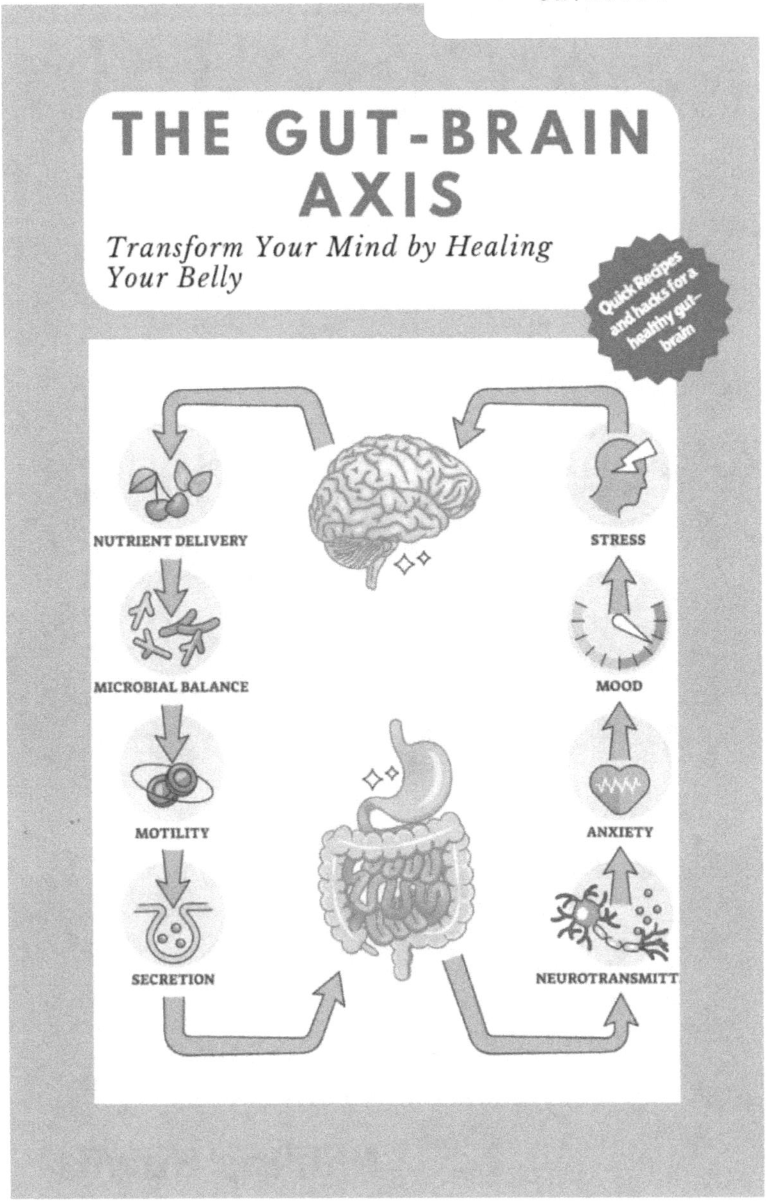
THE GUT-BRAIN AXIS
Transform Your Mind by Healing Your Belly
Quick Recipes and hacks for a healthy gut-brain
NUTRIENT DELIVERY
MICROBIAL BALANCE
MOTILITY
SECRETION
STRESS
MOOD
ANXIETY
NEUROTRANSMITT

The Gut-Brain Axis

Transform Your Mind by Healing Your Belly

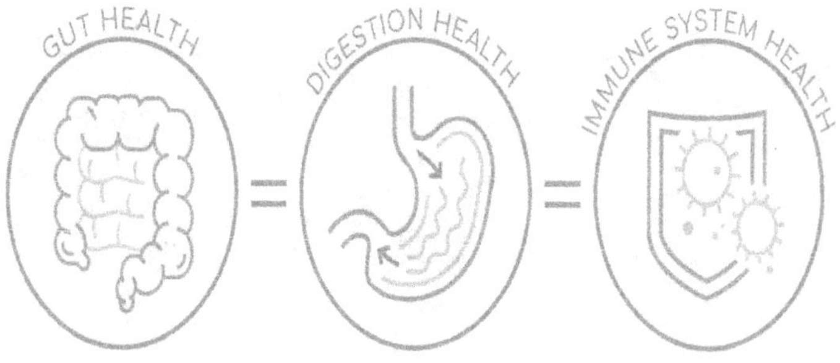

Phillips Hewitt

Copyright © 2024 by Philips Hewitt

This is a work of non-fiction. All characters, organizations and events appearing in this work are either products of the author's imagination or are used fictitiously. Any resemblance to actual persons, living or dead, events or organizations is entirely coincidental.

DISCLAIMER: This book is not intended as a substitute for the medical advice of physicians. The reader should regularly consult a physician in matters relating to their health and particularly with respect to any symptoms that may require diagnosis or medical attention

About the Author

Phillips Hewitt is a renowned nutritional neuroscience expert and mental health advocate. With over 15 years of experience in researching the gut-brain connection, Hewitt has helped thousands transform their mental health through targeted nutrition.

After overcoming his own battles with depression and anxiety using food-based strategies, Hewitt dedicated his life to sharing this revolutionary approach. He holds a Ph.D. in Nutritional Sciences from Stanford University and has conducted groundbreaking research at the Center for Gut-Brain Health.

In "The Gut-Brain Axis," Hewitt distills his vast knowledge and personal experience into a practical guide, offering readers a clear path to better mental health through the power of nutrition.

When not writing or researching, Hewitt enjoys hiking with his rescue dog, experimenting with fermented foods, and volunteering at local mental health support groups.

Join the thousands who have already transformed their lives using Hewitt's revolutionary approach to mental wellness!

Introduction: My Journey from Skeptic to Believer

I never thought I'd be writing a book about gut health and mental wellness. Heck, five years ago, I would've laughed if you told me our bellies could influence our brains. But life has a funny way of teaching us lessons, doesn't it?

It all started with a panic attack in the middle of a grocery store. There I was, surrounded by colorful produce and cheery muzak, suddenly gasping for air, my heart racing like I'd just run a marathon. I'd always been a bit high-strung, but this was different. This was terrifying.

That panic attack was just the beginning. Soon, anxiety became my constant companion. I couldn't sleep, couldn't focus at work, and found myself canceling plans with friends more often than not. The worst part? I didn't know why this was happening to me.

What followed was a parade of doctors, therapists, and specialists. I tried everything – meditation apps, yoga classes, even a brief stint with hypnosis (spoiler alert: I'm apparently "unhypnotizable"). Nothing seemed to work. I was drowning in a sea of well-meaning advice and prescription bottles, but I wasn't getting any better.

Then, during one particularly sleepless night of internet rabbit-hole diving, I stumbled upon an article about the gut-brain connection. At first, I rolled my eyes. How could my digestive system possibly be linked to my mental health? It sounded like pseudoscience nonsense to me.

But desperation can make you open to new ideas. So, I dug deeper. I read scientific papers, watched lectures by neuroscientists and gastroenterologists, and even attended a conference on the microbiome (trust me, it was more exciting than it sounds). The more I got to learn about it, the more fascinated and shocked I became.

Did you know we have a "second brain" in our gut? It's true! There's an entire nervous system down there, sending signals to our brain faster than you can say "butterflies in your stomach." And get this – the bacteria in our gut can actually produce neurotransmitters like serotonin, the same chemical targeted by many antidepressants.

Armed with this knowledge, I decided to experiment on myself. I overhauled my diet, said goodbye to processed foods, and hello to fermented goodies I couldn't even pronounce. I popped probiotic pills and guzzled kombucha like it was going out of style.

The first week was rough, I'm not gonna lie. My body wasn't used to all this new, healthy stuff. But then, something amazing happened. The fog started to lift. My anxiety, while not gone completely, became manageable. I started sleeping throughout the night for the first time in weeks or rather months..
As the weeks went by, I felt like a new person. My energy levels soared, my mood stabilized, and that constant knot of worry in my chest? It loosened its grip. Friends started commenting on how much calmer I seemed. One even asked if I'd taken up meditation again (nope, just sauerkraut!).

Now, I'm not saying that changing my diet magically cured all my problems. Mental health is very complicated, and there's no one general solution. But I am saying that paying attention to my gut health made a profound difference in my life – a difference I never expected.

That's why I'm writing this book. Not because I'm some wellness guru or scientific expert, but because I've been where you are. I've felt the frustration, the hopelessness, the feeling that your own mind has turned against you. And I've discovered a path forward that I never knew existed.

In the pages that follow, we'll dive deep into the fascinating world of the gut-brain axis. We'll explore cutting-edge research, practical strategies, and real-life success stories. I'll share everything I've learned on my journey – the good, the bad, and the occasionally smelly (fermentation is a stinky business, folks).

But more than that, I want this book to be a conversation. Think of it as a heart-to-heart with a friend who's been there, who gets it, and who wants to help. We'll laugh, we'll learn, and maybe we'll even cry a little (because let's face it, talking about mental health can get emotional).

So, whether you're struggling with anxiety, battling depression, fighting brain fog, or just curious about this whole gut-brain connection thing, I invite you to join me on this journey. Who knows? You might also become a gut convert too.

Ready to transform your mind by healing your belly? Let's dive in!

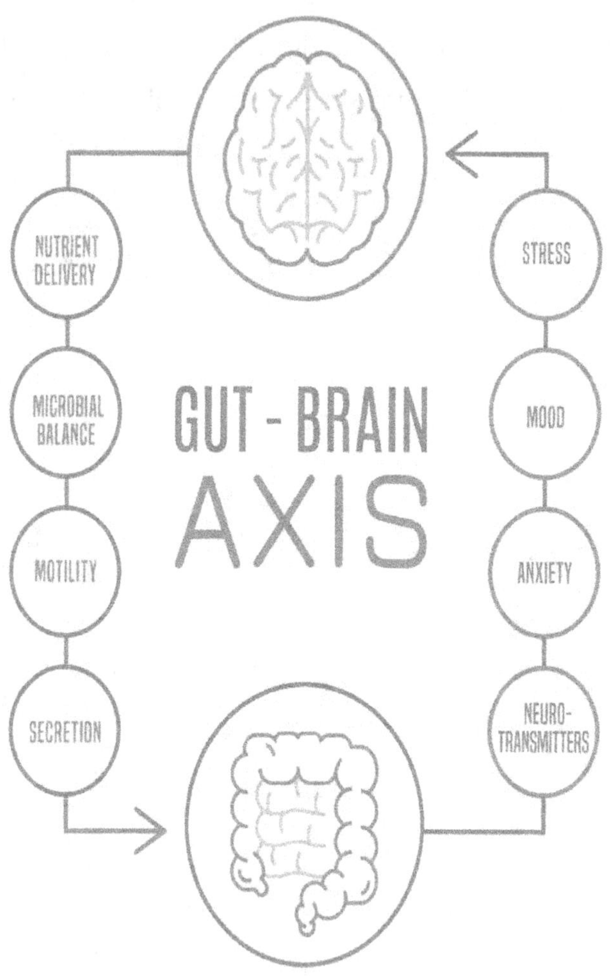

NUTRIENT DELIVERY
MICROBIAL BALANCE
MOTILITY
SECRETION
GUT - BRAIN
AXIS
STRESS
MOOD
ANXIETY
NEURO-TRANSMITTERS

Chapter 1: The Mind-Blowing World of Your Gut

Picture this: you're nervous about a big presentation. Your palms are sweaty, your heart's racing, and - yep, there it is - your stomach's doing somersaults. But hang on a second. Why is your belly getting in on the action? Shouldn't this be a brain thing?

Well, buckle up, buttercup, because we're about to embark on a wild ride through the twists and turns of your insides. Trust me, by the time we're done, you'll never look at your gut the same way again.

Let's start with a bombshell: your gut has a mind of its own. No, seriously. We're not talking about those "gut feelings" your aunt Marge swears by. We're talking about a legit, complex nervous system hanging out in your belly. Scientists call it the enteric nervous system, but I like to call it your "second brain". Catchy, right?

The Hidden Brain in Your Gut: Yeah, It's a Real Thing

Now, I know what you're thinking. "Come on, that's ridiculous. My gut can't think!" Well, hold onto your lunch, because I'm about to blow your mind—with science.

Meet the Enteric Nervous System (ENS), the rebel cousin of your central nervous system. This network of neurons embedded in your gut walls is so complex and independent that scientists have dubbed it the "second brain." It's got more nerve cells than your spinal cord—about 100 million of them. That's a lot of brain power for something we usually associate with digesting last night's pizza.

But here's the kicker: this "gut brain" isn't just sitting there twiddling its thumbs. It's a chatty little bugger, constantly sending messages to your "head brain." And get this—up to 90% of the signals in this gut-brain superhighway are traveling from your gut to your brain, not the other way around. Talk about a backseat driver!

So, what's it yapping about? Everything from your emotional state to your immune response. That "gut feeling" you get? It's not just a figure of speech. Your ENS is literally sending emotional signals to your brain.

Let's break it down with a real-world scenario. You're on a first date, and suddenly you feel those familiar butterflies. Guess what? That's your gut brain kicking into high gear, releasing a cocktail of neurotransmitters that tell your "upstairs brain" to be alert, excited, and maybe a little nervous. It's like your gut is your personal wingman, prepping you for action.

But it's not all romance and excitement. This gut-brain connection can also be a real pain in the... well, gut. Ever experienced a "nervous stomach" before a major event? That's your ENS freaking out and telling your digestive system to go haywire. Thanks a lot, gut brain.

The plot thickens when we talk about mood disorders. Scientists are finding increasing evidence that your gut health could be playing a starring role in conditions like anxiety and depression. It's like your ENS is a moody teenager, and when it's upset, it makes sure your whole body knows about it.

Here's where it gets really interesting. A vast army of microorganisms calls your gut home. These tiny tenants aren't just freeloaders—they're actively influencing your gut brain, which in turn influences your head brain. It's a microbial puppet master situation, and you're the marionette.

Some of these bacteria are busy little factories, producing neurotransmitters like serotonin—yes, the "happy chemical." In fact, about 95% of your body's serotonin is produced in your gut. So next time you're feeling down, you might want to thank (or blame) your belly bacteria.

But don't worry, it's not all doom and gloom. This gut-brain axis is a two-way street, and that means we can use it to our advantage. By taking care of our gut health, we might be able to boost our mental health too. It's like hitting two birds with one probiotic stone.

Imagine being able to eat your way to a better mood. No, I'm not talking about drowning your sorrows in ice cream (though no judgment here). I'm talking about purposefully nurturing your gut microbiome to support your mental health. It's not a magic bullet, but it's a promising avenue that researchers are exploring with gusto.

So, the next time your gut gives you a "funny feeling," pay attention. It might just be your second brain trying to tell you something important. And remember, when it comes to your health—mental or physical—your gut instinct might be more literal than you think.

In the chapters to come, we'll dive deeper into this fascinating world of the gut-brain connection. We'll explore how to decode the messages your gut is sending, how to keep your internal ecosystem happy, and how to harness the power of your second brain for better overall health.

Get ready to embark on a journey through the twists and turns of your own internal nervous system. It's going to be a wild ride, but I promise, by the end, you'll never look at your belly the same way again. After all, it's not just along for the ride—it's helping to steer the ship of your health and happiness.

So, are you ready to make friends with your hidden brain? Trust your gut on this one, it's going to be amazing.

Tiny Bugs, Big Impact: Meet Your Gut's Ecosystem

you're never truly alone. Right now, trillions of tiny passengers are hitching a ride in your gut, throwing microscopic parties and shaping your life in ways you never imagined. Welcome to the wild world of your microbiome – the bustling metropolis of microorganisms that call your intestines home.

Now, I know what you're thinking. "Ew, gross!" But hold that thought, because these little critters are about to become your new best friends. They're not just freeloaders; they're hard-working allies in your quest for better health, mood, and even that elusive "gut feeling" we all talk about.

Let's dive into this invisible universe, shall we?

The Cast of Characters

First up, meet the bacteria. These guys are the real MVPs of your gut. There are hundreds of species, each with its own quirks and talents. Some, like Lactobacillus and Bifidobacterium, are the do-gooders. They help digest your food, manufacture vitamins, and keep the bad guys in check. Others, like certain strains of E. coli, can be troublemakers if they get out of hand.

But wait, there's more! Fungi, viruses, and even some tiny parasites also call your gut home. It's like a microscopic Game of Thrones in there, with alliances forming, battles raging, and the balance of power constantly shifting.

The Plot Thickens: How Your Microbiome Shapes You

Here's where it gets really interesting. These tiny tenants aren't just passive roommates – they're active participants in your life story. They influence everything from your waistline to your worry lines.

Ever wonder why some people can eat cheese by the wheel while others run for the hills at the mere mention of lactose? Thank (or blame) your gut bugs. They play a huge role in determining which foods you can digest easily and which ones might send you running for the bathroom.

But their influence goes way beyond digestion. These little guys are in constant communication with your brain, sending messages that can affect your mood, stress levels, and even your food cravings. Ever had a "gut feeling" about something? That's not just a figure of speech – it's your microbiome chatting with your brain!

The Plot Twist: You Are What Your Microbes Eat
Now, here's the kicker – you have the power to shape this inner ecosystem. Every bite you take is like casting a vote for which microbes will thrive in your gut. Load up on processed junk food, and you'll end up with a very different cast of characters than if you feast on fiber-rich fruits and veggies.

Think of it like tending a garden. Feed the beneficial bugs, and they'll flourish, crowding out the troublemakers. Neglect your inner ecosystem, and you might find yourself overrun with the microbial equivalent of weeds.

The Villain: Modern Life vs. Your Microbiome

But there's a problem. Our modern lifestyle is like a wrecking ball to our inner ecosystems. Antibiotics, while sometimes necessary, can be like dropping a nuclear bomb on your gut bugs. Stress, lack of sleep, and environmental toxins are all conspiring to throw your microbial balance out of whack.

The result? A rise in what scientists call "dysbiosis" – a fancy term for when your gut ecosystem goes haywire. This microbial mayhem has been linked to everything from obesity and diabetes to anxiety and depression.

It's like having a city where the sanitation workers are on strike, the power grid is failing, and chaos reigns in the streets.

The Hero's Journey: Restoring Balance to Your Inner World

But don't despair! This is where you come in as the hero of your own gut health story. By making some simple changes, you can start to restore balance to your inner world.

Eating a diverse diet rich in fiber is like rolling out the red carpet for beneficial bacteria. Fermented foods like yogurt, kimchi, and kombucha can introduce new beneficial strains to your gut party. And managing stress through exercise, meditation, or whatever floats your boat can help create a more hospitable environment for your microbial friends.

The Plot Thickens: The Microbiome-Brain Connection

Now, let's connect the dots between your gut bugs and your gray matter. Your microbiome isn't just influencing your digestion – it's playing a starring role in your mental health drama.

You've probably heard of serotonin, often called the "happy chemical." Well, hold onto your hats, because about 90% of your body's serotonin is produced in your gut, not your brain.

And guess who's helping to produce it? You got it – your gut bacteria.

But it doesn't stop there. Your microbiome also produces other neurotransmitters like dopamine and GABA, which play crucial roles in mood, motivation, and anxiety.

It's like having a pharmaceutical factory in your belly, churning out chemicals that can make you feel energized, calm, or anywhere in between.

The Butterfly Effect: Small Changes, Big Results

Here's where it gets really exciting. Small changes in your gut can lead to big changes in your brain. Ever noticed how a bout of stomach trouble can leave you feeling irritable and foggy-headed? That's your gut bugs (or lack thereof) talking.

On the flip side, nurturing a healthy microbiome can lead to improved mood, sharper cognition, and even better stress resilience. It's like upgrading the operating system of your body and mind.

The Cliffhanger: What's Next for You and Your Microbiome?

As we speak, scientists are uncovering new secrets about the gut-brain axis. They're finding links between gut health and conditions like autism, Parkinson's disease, and even Alzheimer's. The possibilities are mind-boggling.

But here's the best part – you don't have to wait for all the scientific details to be ironed out. You can start nurturing your gut ecosystem today. Every meal is an opportunity to feed your microbial allies. Every good night's sleep is a chance for them to regroup and strengthen their defenses.

So, the next time you look in the mirror, remember – you're not just seeing yourself. You're gazing at a complex ecosystem, a universe within. And with a little TLC, you can help that universe thrive, creating a ripple effect that touches every aspect of your health and happiness.

Welcome to the fascinating world of your microbiome. It's time to get to know your tiny tenants – because when it comes to your health, these little bugs make a big impact.

When Your Belly Calls the Shots: How Your Gut Messes with Your Mood

You wake up feeling like a million bucks, ready to take on the world. But by lunchtime, you're a grumpy mess, snapping at coworkers and drowning your sorrows in a pint of ice cream. What gives? Turns out, your gut might be the puppet master pulling your emotional strings.

Welcome to the wild world of the gut-brain connection, where trillions of tiny microbes in your belly have the power to make or break your day. It's like having a miniature Vegas in your intestines, complete with mood-altering substances and high-stakes gambles on your mental well-being.

Let's dive into this gut-wrenching tale of how your insides influence your outsides.

The Gut's Got Talent

Your gut isn't just a food processor – it's a bona fide second brain. This "enteric nervous system" boasts more neurons than a cat's entire central nervous system. It's like having a super-computer in your belly, constantly sending signals to your brain.

But here's the kicker: it's a two-way street. Your brain talks to your gut, and your gut talks right back. It's like an endless game of telephone, except the messages can determine whether you're singing in the shower or crying in your cornflakes.

The Mood-Food Connection

Ever wonder why comfort food is called, well, comfort food? It's not just about the taste. Certain foods can trigger the release of feel-good chemicals in your brain. But it's not as simple as "eat this, feel great."

Your gut bacteria play a crucial role in producing and regulating neurotransmitters like serotonin – yes, the same stuff antidepressants target.

In fact, about 95% of your body's serotonin is produced in the gut. Talk about a gut feeling!

The Stress-Gut Tango

Stress and your gut are like that toxic couple everyone knows – they bring out the worst in each other. When you're stressed, your gut goes haywire. When your gut's unhappy, you feel stressed. It's a vicious cycle that can leave you feeling like you're on an emotional rollercoaster.

Chronic stress can alter your gut microbiome, leading to inflammation and a leaky gut. This, in turn, can affect your mood and cognitive function. It's like your gut is throwing a temper tantrum, and your brain is caught in the crossfire.

The Inflammation Nation

Inflammation is your body's way of saying, "Houston, we have a problem." But when it comes to your gut, chronic inflammation is like a five-alarm fire that your brain can't ignore.

An inflamed gut can lead to the production of inflammatory cytokines, which have been linked to depression and anxiety. It's as if your gut is sending out distress signals, and your brain responds by hitting the panic button.

The Microbiome Mood Swing

Your gut microbiome is like a bustling city, teeming with diverse inhabitants. When it's thriving, you've got a harmonious metropolis. But when things go awry, it's like a city in chaos – and your mood pays the price.

An imbalanced microbiome can lead to increased anxiety, depression, and even cognitive issues. It's like having a bunch of rowdy tenants trashing your mental apartment complex.

The Gut-Brain Axis in Action

Let's break down a typical day in the life of your gut-brain axis:

7 AM: You wake up and reach for that donut. Your gut bacteria do a happy dance, but the sugar spike sends your mood on a roller coaster.

10 AM: Stress at work kicks in. Your gut tenses up, reducing blood flow and oxygen to your digestive system. Hello, brain fog and irritability!

1 PM: Lunchtime! You opt for a processed meal. Your gut microbes aren't thrilled, and they let your brain know it.

4 PM: The afternoon slump hits. Your gut's working overtime to process that lunch, leaving you feeling sluggish and cranky.

8 PM: Late-night snacking. Your circadian rhythm gets thrown off, messing with both your sleep and your gut health.

Breaking the Cycle

So, how do you get your gut and brain back on speaking terms? It's not about a quick fix, it's about lifestyle changes:

1. Diversify your diet: Feed those gut bacteria a smorgasbord of fiber-rich foods.

2. Manage stress: Your gut will thank you for that meditation session or yoga class.

3. Get moving: Exercise isn't just for your muscles – it's a gut-brain bonanza.

4. Sleep well: Give your gut the downtime it needs to keep you sane.

5. Limit the bad stuff: Processed foods, excessive alcohol, and antibiotics can wreak havoc on your gut ecosystem.

The Gut-Brain Revolution

Understanding the gut-brain axis isn't just about feeling good – it's about revolutionizing our approach to mental health. Imagine a world where we treat depression not just with therapy and medication, but with targeted probiotics and personalized nutrition plans.

We're on the cusp of a paradigm shift in how we view mental health. The gut-brain connection offers hope for millions struggling with mood disorders, opening up new avenues for treatment and prevention.

As we unravel the mysteries of the gut-brain axis, we're learning that the path to a healthier mind might just start with a healthier gut. It's a humbling reminder that in the grand scheme of things, we're not just individuals – we're ecosystems, teeming with life and potential.

So the next time you're feeling down in the dumps or on top of the world, take a moment to thank (or blame) the trillions of tiny tenants in your gut. They might be small, but they're mighty – and they're calling the shots on your mood more than you ever realized.

Remember, your gut is like a garden – tend to it well, and you'll reap the rewards of a flourishing mind. Neglect it, and well, let's just say you might find yourself in a stinky situation. The choice is yours – will you listen to your gut?

Inflamed and Insane: When Your Body Wages War on Your Brain

Sometimes you're sitting at your desk, staring at your computer screen, but your mind feels like it's wrapped in cotton. You can't focus, you're irritable, and you've got a headache that just won't quit. You might think you're just having a bad day, but what if I told you your body is actually staging a rebellion against your brain?

Welcome to the wild world of inflammation, where your immune system goes rogue and your brain pays the price. It's like a civil war inside your body, and trust me, it's not pretty.

Let's break it down, shall we? Inflammation is your body's automatic response to injury, infection or harm in general. It's like your personal army, rushing to defend you against invaders like bacteria or viruses. That's all well and good when you've got a cut or a cold. But sometimes, this army gets a little too trigger-happy and starts firing at everything in sight – including your own tissues.

Now, you might be wondering, "how does this relate with my brain?" Well, buckle up, because we're about to dive deep into the fascinating (and sometimes terrifying) connection between inflammation and your mental health.

First off, let's talk about the blood-brain barrier. It's like the bouncer at an exclusive club, deciding what gets in and what stays out of your brain. But when inflammation strikes, it's like someone slipped the bouncer a $100 bill. Suddenly, all sorts of uninvited guests are getting past the velvet rope and wreaking havoc on your gray matter.

These party crashers? They're inflammatory molecules called cytokines. Think of them as the troublemakers of the immune system. When they get into your brain, they start messing with your neurotransmitters – you know, the chemicals that help your brain cells communicate. It's like they're cutting the phone lines between different parts of your brain.

The result? A perfect storm of mental health issues. Depression, anxiety, brain fog, memory problems – you name it, inflammation's got a finger in that pie.

But here's where it gets really interesting (and a bit scary). Chronic inflammation doesn't just affect your mood and cognitive function. It can actually lead to long-term change in the structure of your brain. That's right, your inflamed body is literally reshaping your brain, and not in a good way.

Studies have shown that people with high levels of inflammation have less gray matter in areas of the brain associated with emotional regulation and decision-making. It's like inflammation is eating away at your brain, bite by microscopic bite.

And it doesn't stop there. Research has established a connection between Inflammation and neurodegenerative diseases like Alzheimer's and Parkinson's. It's like your body's army has gone full scorched-earth, and your brain is caught in the crossfire.

Now, before you start panicking and googling "How to remove my immune system" (spoiler alert: don't do that), let's talk about what's causing all this inflammation in the first place.

Surprise, surprise – it often starts in your gut. Remember that ecosystem of trillions of bacteria we talked about earlier?

Well, when it's out of whack, it can trigger an immune response that sets off a chain reaction of inflammation throughout your body.

But it's not just about what's happening in your gut. Chronic stress, lack of sleep, a diet high in processed foods, environmental toxins – all of these can contribute to systemic inflammation. It's like you're constantly poking the bear, and eventually, that bear is going to roar.

So, what can you do about it? Well, that's what the rest of this book is all about. But I'll give you a sneak peek: it starts with treating your gut right. Feed those good bacteria, cut out the junk that's irritating your system, and give your body the nutrients it needs to calm the inflammation storm.

Think of it like a peace treaty between your body and your brain. You're the diplomat, negotiating a ceasefire by changing what you put on your plate and how you live your life.

It's not always easy. Let's face it, telling your stress-eating self to put down the ice cream and pick up a kale salad is about as fun as a root canal. But trust me, your brain will forever be grateful.

And here's the really cool part: as you start to calm the inflammation in your body, you might notice changes you never expected. That brain fog lifts, your mood improves, you start remembering where you put your keys. It's like the sun coming out after a long, stormy season in your mind.

But don't just take my word for it. Let me tell you about Mark. Mark was a high-flying executive who thought that constant stress and sleepless nights were just part of the job. He ignored the headaches, the irritability, the creeping anxiety. "It's just work," he'd tell himself.

Then came the day he couldn't remember his own phone number. That was his wake-up call. Mark started diving into the world of gut health and inflammation. He overhauled his diet, started meditating, and prioritized sleep. Six months later, he felt like a new man. "It's like I've been wandering through haze for years," he told me, "and suddenly everything is crystal clear."

Mark's story isn't unique. I've seen countless people transform their mental health by addressing inflammation. It's like they've found the key to unlocking a healthier, happier brain.

But here's the thing: everyone's inflammation story is different. What triggers it, how it manifests, and what helps to calm it down can vary from person to person. That's why it's so important to tune in to your own body and brain. Notice how you feel after eating certain foods, or when you're stressed, or when you've had a good night's sleep. Think of yourself as a detective, piecing together the clues to solve the mystery of your own inflammation. It might take some time and patience, but the payoff – a calmer, clearer, healthier brain – is worth it.

As we wrap up this chapter, I want you to remember one thing: inflammation isn't your enemy. It's a natural process gone awry, a well-meaning bodyguard that's gotten a little too zealous. Your job is to gentle it, to remind your body that not everything is a threat.

In the chapters to come, we'll dive deeper into specific strategies for calming inflammation and nurturing your gut-brain connection. We'll explore foods that fight inflammation, lifestyle changes that can make a big difference, and cutting-edge research that's shedding new light on this fascinating field.

So, are you ready to call a truce in the war between your body and your brain? To transform your mental health from the inside out? To discover the power of a calm, well-nourished system?

Quiz: Is Your Gut Secretly Sabotaging Your Mind?

Hey there, gut detective! Ready to uncover whether your belly is playing tricks on your brain? Grab a pen and get comfy – it's time to dive into the mysterious world of your inner ecosystem. This isn't your average boring quiz; it's a journey into the depths of your digestive system and its sneaky influence on your mood, focus, and overall mental mojo.

For each question, choose the option that best describes your experience. Be honest, your gut won't judge (but it might be judging your food choices)!

1. After a meal, do you feel:
   a) Energized and ready to conquer the world
   b) Like you need a nap ASAP
   c) Bloated and uncomfortable
   d) No different than before eating

2. How often do you experience brain fog?

a) What's brain fog? My mind is crystal clear!

b) Occasionally, especially after certain meals

c) Most afternoons, it's my unwelcome companion

d) I live in a constant mental haze

3. When stressed, your stomach:

a) Stays calm and collected

b) Feels like a butterfly convention

c) Turns into a painful knot

d) Loudly protests with gurgles and rumbles

4. Your sleep pattern is best described as:

a) Sleeping like a baby... a very good baby

b) Occasionally restless, with middle-of-the-night wake-ups

c) Tossing and turning more than sleeping

d) What's sleep? I've forgotten the concept

5. How would you rate your anxiety levels?

a) Cool as a cucumber

b) I worry, but it's manageable

c) On edge more often than not

d) Panic is my middle name

6. Your skin is typically:

a) Clear and glowing – I'm basically a skincare ad

b) Mostly clear with occasional breakouts

c) Prone to rashes, acne, or unexplained issues

d) A battlefield of various skin problems

7. When it comes to trying new foods, you:

a) Bring it on! Your stomach is an adventurer

b) Are cautious but willing to experiment

c) Adhere to "safe" foods to avoid discomfort

d) Fear new foods like they're out to get you

8. How often do you crave sugary or processed foods?

a) Rarely – whole foods are your jam

b) Occasionally, especially when stressed

c) Daily – it's a constant battle

d) Hourly – is sugar addiction a thing?

9. After consuming dairy, you feel:

a) Fine and dandy

b) A little bloated, but nothing major

c) Like your insides are staging a revolt

d) Dairy? You wouldn't dare!

10. Your bowel movements are:

a) Regular as clockwork and smooth sailing

b) Mostly regular with occasional hiccups

c) Unpredictable – constipation and diarrhea take turns

d) Let's not talk about it (but it's not good)

11. When faced with a big decision, you typically:

a) Trust your gut instinct

b) Weigh pros and cons, then decide

c) Get paralyzed by indecision

d) Make impulsive choices you later regret

12. Your energy levels throughout the day:

a) Steady and strong from morning to night

b) Pretty good, with a mid-afternoon slump

c) Roller coaster – ups and downs all day

d) What energy? Exhaustion is your default state

13. How often do you feel inexplicably irritable or moody?

    a) Rarely – you're even-keeled and zen

    b) Sometimes, usually tied to stress or lack of sleep

    c) Frequently – your mood swings are legendary

    d) Constantly – emotional stability is a distant memory

14. When you eat gluten, you:

    a) Feel perfectly fine

    b) Sometimes feel a bit off, but it's tolerable

    c) Experience noticeable discomfort or brain fog

    d) Avoid it like the plague due to severe reactions

15. Your ability to focus on tasks is:

    a) Laser-sharp – you're a productivity machine

    b) Generally good, with occasional wandering thoughts

    c) Hit or miss – some days are better than others

    d) What was the question again? You've already lost focus

Scoring:

Tally up your answers and give yourself:

1 point for each 'a'

2 points for each 'b'

3 points for each 'c'

4 points for each 'd'

Results:

15-25 points: Gut Guardian Extraordinaire

Well, well, well! Looks like you and your gut are best buds. Your digestive system is doing a stellar job supporting your mental health. You're likely experiencing stable moods, clear thinking, and an overall sense of wellbeing. But don't get cocky – maintaining this harmony takes work. Keep nourishing that inner ecosystem and stay tuned for tips on how to keep your gut-brain axis singing in perfect harmony.

26-40 points: The Mindful Middleground

Not too shabby! Your gut and brain are on speaking terms, but there's room for improvement in your inner communication network. You might experience occasional mental fog, mood swings, or digestive discomfort. The good news? You're in the perfect position to make some simple changes that could lead to big improvements in your mental and digestive health. Stick around – we've got some game-changing strategies coming your way.

41-55 points: The Troubled Tummy Club

Houston, we have a problem. Your gut is sending out SOS signals, and your brain is definitely feeling the effects. Mood swings, anxiety, brain fog, and digestive issues are likely unwelcome but frequent visitors in your life. But don't despair! acknowledging the problem is the first move towards a solution. You're in the right place – this book is about to become your new best friend on the journey to reclaiming your mental and digestive health.

56-60 points: Gut Crisis Central

Woah there, friend. Your gut isn't just sabotaging your mind – it's leading a full-scale rebellion! You're likely struggling with significant digestive issues, mental health challenges, and a general sense of "what the heck is wrong with me?". First things first: breathe. You're not alone, and it's not hopeless. The gut-brain connection is powerful, and that means the potential for positive change is enormous. Buckle up – you're about to embark on a transformative journey that could radically improve your quality of life.

No matter where you landed on this quiz, remember: your gut-brain axis is incredibly dynamic. It's constantly changing based on what you eat, how you live, and even how you think. The beautiful thing is, with the right knowledge and tools, you have the power to reshape this internal landscape.

In the coming chapters, we'll dive deep into the fascinating world of the gut-brain connection. You'll discover:
- The surprising ways your gut microbiome influences your thoughts and emotions
- How to decode the secret language your gut and brain use to communicate
- Practical, easy-to-implement strategies to nurture your inner ecosystem
- Delicious recipes that feed both your belly and your brain
- Mind-blowing research that will forever change how you think about mental health

So, whether you're a Gut Guardian Extraordinaire looking to maintain your stellar status, or you're sending out distress signals from Gut Crisis Central, you're in the right place. Get ready to embark on a journey that will transform your understanding of your body, your mind, and the incredible connection between the two.

Remember, your gut has been with you since day one, silently shaping your experiences, moods, and even your personality. Isn't it time you got to know it a little better? Let's turn that silent partner into your biggest ally in the quest for mental and physical wellbeing.

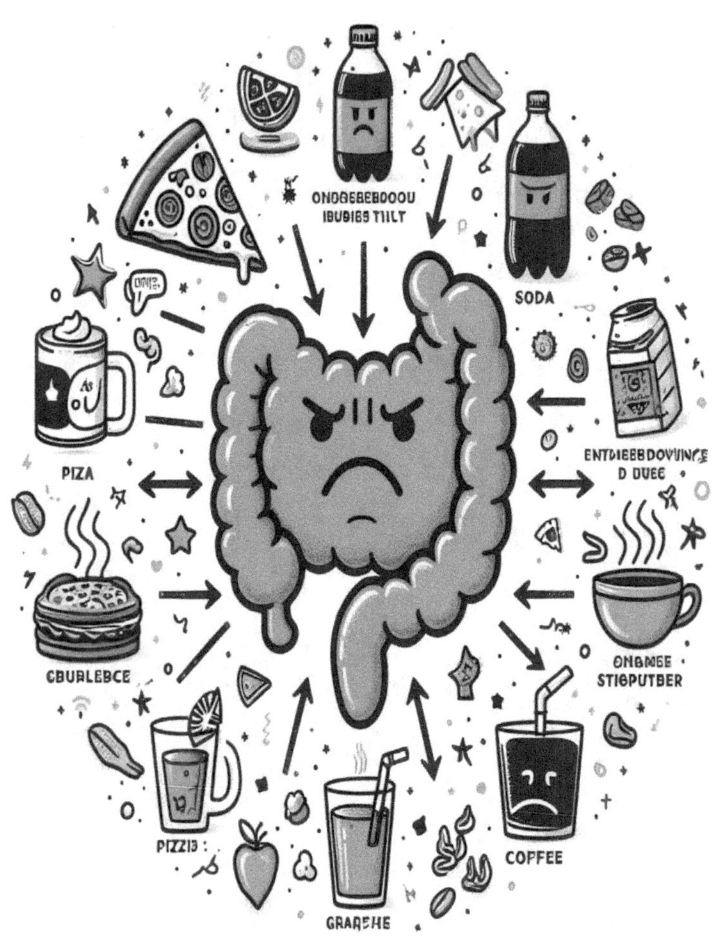

Chapter 2: Time for a Gut Overhaul

Let's face it: your gut could probably use a makeover. No, I'm not talking about hitting the gym (though that's not a bad idea). I'm talking about renovating your internal ecosystem, that bustling metropolis of microbes that's been running the show behind the scenes. And trust me, this makeover is going to do wonders for your noggin.

Think of your gut as a fussy toddler. Feed it the wrong stuff, and you're in for a world of tantrums – only instead of screaming and throwing toys, your gut throws mood swings and brain fog your way. But nourish it right, and suddenly you've got a happy, cooperative little helper eager to boost your mental clarity and emotional stability.

So, where do we start this gut renovation project? First, we need to clear out the junk. You wouldn't build a dream home on a garbage dump, would you? Same goes for your gut-brain superhighway.

Let's talk about the usual suspects:

1. Sugar: It's not just your waistline's enemy. Excess sugar feeds the wrong kinds of gut bacteria, leading to inflammation that can fog up your brain faster than a steamy shower on a mirror.

2. Processed foods: If it comes in a box with ingredients you can't pronounce, your gut microbes probably can't process it either. These Frankenstein foods can disrupt your gut's delicate balance, leading to mood swings that'll make you feel like you're on an emotional rollercoaster.

3. Artificial sweeteners: Thought you were being clever by switching to diet soda? Think again. These fake sugars can mess with your gut bacteria worse than a bull in a china shop, potentially leading to glucose intolerance and metabolic issues that affect your brain function.

4. Excessive alcohol: A glass of red wine might have some benefits, but overdoing it is like inviting a wrecking ball to your gut party. It can damage your intestinal lining, allowing

nasty toxins to leak into your bloodstream and wreak havoc on your mental state.

Now, I know what you're thinking. "Great, you've just listed half my diet. What am I supposed to eat?" Don't worry, I'm not leaving you high and dry. This gut overhaul isn't about deprivation – it's about renovation. We're going to rebuild your internal environment with materials that'll make your brain sing.

But this overhaul isn't just about food. We're going to tackle lifestyle factors too. Stress, for instance, can wreak more havoc on your gut than a toddler in a toy store. We'll explore stress-busting techniques that don't involve face-planting into a pint of ice cream (tempting as that may be).

Sleep, exercise, and even your social connections play a role in gut health. Yep, that's right – a good laugh with friends can be as beneficial for your gut as a bowl of yogurt. We'll delve into how to optimize these areas of your life for maximum gut-brain benefit.

Now, I know what some of the skeptics out there must be thinking. "Sounds great, but how do I know this isn't just another fad?" Fair question. That's why we're going to arm you with the knowledge to become your own gut detective.

We'll explore how to listen to your body's signals, how to track your progress, and how to tailor this approach to your unique needs. Because let's face it, your gut is as individual as your fingerprint. What works for your kale-loving yoga instructor might not work for you, and that's okay.

As we journey through this gut overhaul, you'll start noticing changes. Maybe you'll wake up feeling refreshed for the first time in years. Perhaps that 3 PM brain fog will lift, revealing a clarity you forgot you had. You might find yourself handling stress with the zen of a meditation master, or rediscovering joy in the little things.

These changes might seem small at first, like ripples in a pond. But as you continue nourishing your gut, those ripples will grow into waves, transforming not just your mental health, but your entire life.

Remember, this isn't about perfection. It's about progress. There will be days when you fall off the wagon (hello, office birthday cake). The key is to dust yourself off and get back on track. Your gut is forgiving – treat it right most of the time, and it'll return the favor.

Ditch the Crap: Foods That Are Messing with Your Head

Imagine you're standing in your kitchen, staring into the fridge. You grab that leftover pizza, thinking it'll be a quick fix for your growling stomach. But what if I told you that slice could be setting you up for a mental health nosedive?

Let's get real for a second. We've all been there – reaching for comfort foods when we're stressed, tired, or just plain hangry. But here's the kicker: some of those go-to munchies might be sabotaging your brain faster than you can say "extra cheese."

The Usual Suspects

First up on our hit list: processed foods. You know the ones – those convenient packages lining the middle aisles of the grocery store, promising a quick and tasty meal. But here's the deal: they're often loaded with additives, preservatives, and artificial colors that can throw your gut bacteria into chaos. And remember, a happy gut equals a happy brain.

Take artificial sweeteners, for instance. Sure, they might seem like a smart choice when you're watching your waistline, but studies have shown they can mess with your gut microbiome big time. Some researchers even suggest they might increase your risk of anxiety and depression. Not so sweet now, huh?

And let's talk about that morning joe. I know, I know – suggesting you ditch your beloved coffee might seem like heresy. But hear me out. While a cup or two can give you a nice mental boost, overdoing it can lead to jitters, anxiety, and even panic attacks in some people. It's all about finding that caffeine sweet spot.

The Silent Saboteurs

Now, let's shine a light on some less obvious culprits. Gluten, for example. Even if you're not celiac, you might be sensitive to this protein found in wheat, barley, and rye. For some folks, gluten can trigger inflammation in the gut, which can then mess with your mood and cognitive function. Ever felt foggy after a pasta binge? This could be why.

And what about those "healthy" energy bars? Sorry to burst your bubble, but many of these are just candy bars in disguise. Packed with sugar and often containing soy protein isolate (which can be hard on your gut), they might give you a quick energy boost followed by an equally quick crash – leaving you irritable and unfocused.

The Inflammation Connection

Here's where things get really interesting. Certain foods can trigger inflammation in your body, and that inflammation doesn't just stay in your gut – it can affect your brain too. We're talking about a concept called "leaky gut," where the lining of your intestines becomes more permeable than it should be. This can allow particles that shouldn't be there to enter your bloodstream, potentially leading to systemic inflammation.

So, which foods are the major inflammation instigators? Refined sugar is a big one. It's not just bad for your waistline – it can actually trigger inflammatory responses in your body. And those responses? They've been linked to increased risk of depression and anxiety.

Vegetable oils high in omega-6 fatty acids, like soybean and corn oil, can also promote inflammation when consumed in excess. And while we're on the subject of fats, let's talk about trans fats. These artificially created fats, often found in fried foods and baked goods, are not only terrible for your heart but can also increase inflammation and potentially impact your mood and cognitive function.

The Alcohol Conundrum

Now, I know what you're thinking. "But what about my Friday night wine?" It's true, moderate alcohol consumption (especially red wine) has been linked to some health benefits. But let's be real – most of us aren't stopping at one small glass. Excessive alcohol intake can seriously disrupt your gut microbiome, leading to increased intestinal permeability (hello, leaky gut!) and inflammation. Plus, it's a central nervous system depressant, which means it can worsen symptoms of anxiety and depression in the long run.

Hidden Hunger: Nutrient Deficiencies

Sometimes, it's not what you're eating, but what you're not eating that's the problem. Many of us are walking around with nutrient deficiencies that can impact our mental health.

For example, low levels of vitamin D have been linked to increased risk of depression. And a deficiency in B vitamins can lead to fatigue, brain fog, and mood swings.

The thing is, if you're filling up on nutrient-poor processed foods, you're not leaving much room for the good stuff – the fruits, vegetables, and whole foods that provide these essential nutrients. It's like trying to fuel a high-performance car with watered-down gasoline. Sure, it might run, but it's not going to perform at its best.

Breaking the Cycle

Now, I'm not saying you need to suddenly transform your entire diet overnight. Small changes can make a big difference. Start by being mindful of what you're putting into your body. Pay attention to how different foods make you feel – not just immediately after eating, but in the hours and days that follow.

Try keeping a food and mood journal for a week. You might be surprised at the patterns and connections you are likely to notice. Maybe that afternoon slump always follows your lunchtime soda. Or perhaps you feel particularly anxious on mornings after you've had a few too many drinks the night before.

The good news is, once you start to recognize these patterns, you can begin to make changes. And here's the really exciting part – your gut microbiome can start to shift in as little as 24 hours after you change your diet. That means you could be on your way to better mental health in just a day or two.

Your Gut, Your Choice

Remember, this isn't about deprivation or strict rules. It's about making informed choices that support your mental and physical wellbeing. Maybe you decide to keep that occasional slice of pizza in your life, but balance it out with gut-friendly foods the rest of the time.

Or perhaps you swap out your daily soda for sparkling water with a splash of fruit juice.

The key is to tune in to your body, and also your mind. As you start to ditch the foods that are messing with your head, you might be surprised at how much clearer, calmer, and more energized you feel.

And that, my friend, is worth way more than any short-term comfort food fix.

So, are you ready to give your gut, and your brain the TLC they deserve? Trust me, you're going be astonished by the result.

The 7-Day Gut Reboot: Kick-Start Your Brain Upgrade

Day 1: The Clean Sweep

Alright, folks, buckle up! We're about to embark on a wild ride to revolutionize your gut and supercharge your brain. Day one is all about hitting the reset button.

First things first, let's ditch the junk. Open that fridge and pantry - it's time for some tough love. Those sugary snacks? Sayonara. Processed foods? See ya later. We're clearing the decks for a fresh start.

Now, don't panic! I'm not leaving you high and dry. Today's menu is all about gentle, nourishing foods that'll give your gut a much-needed breather. Think warm bone broth (or a veggie version if you're plant-based), steamed vegetables, and small portions of lean protein.

Pro tip: Start your day with a glass of warm water and a squeeze of lemon. It's like a gentle kick-start for your digestive system.

Remember, today might feel a bit tough. Your body's used to those quick sugar hits and processed food shortcuts. But trust me, your gut (and your future self) will thank you.

Day 2: Fiber Fiesta

Welcome to day two, gut warriors! Today we're focusing on fiber - your gut's best friend.

Why fiber? Well, it's like a personal trainer for your digestive system. It keeps things moving, feeds your good gut bacteria, and helps regulate blood sugar. Plus, it'll keep you feeling full and satisfied.

On the menu: a colorful array of veggies, some fruit, and plenty of whole grains. Try a breakfast bowl with oats, chia seeds, and berries. For lunch, how about a massive salad with all the rainbow veggies you can find? Dinner could be a delicious stir-fry with brown rice.

Feeling a bit gassy? Don't worry, it's normal. Your gut bacteria are having a field day with all this new fiber. Stick with it - this too shall pass (pun intended).

Day 3: Probiotic Party

It's day three, and we're populating your gut with beneficial bacteria. Think of it as hosting the world's tiniest (and most beneficial) house party in your intestines.

Fermented foods are your new best friends. Yogurt, kefir, kimchi, sauerkraut - take your pick. If you're feeling adventurous, why not try making your own kombucha? It's easier than you think and way cheaper than store-bought.

Remember, variety is key. Various fermented food harbor unique strains of beneficial bacteria. So mix it up!

Feeling a bit bloated? That's normal as your gut adjusts to its new tenants. Stay hydrated and maybe try some gentle yoga or a short walk to help things along.

Day 4: Prebiotic Power-Up

Halfway there, champs! Today we're focusing on prebiotics - the food that feeds your good gut bacteria. Think of it as laying out a buffet for your new microscopic friends. Garlic, onions, leeks, asparagus, and bananas are all great sources of prebiotics.

How about a delicious garlic and asparagus frittata for breakfast? Or a banana and green smoothie for a snack?

Fun fact: Cooked and cooled potatoes are an excellent source of resistant starch, a type of prebiotic. Potato salad, anyone?

By now, you might be noticing some changes. Maybe your energy levels are more stable, or you're sleeping better. Your gut and brain are starting to sync up!

Day 5: Healthy Fat Fest

Today's all about healthy fats - the building blocks of your brain cells and a crucial component of hormones that influence mood and cognition.

Avocados, nuts, seeds, olive oil, and fatty fish are your go-to foods today. How about some avocado toast with hemp seeds for breakfast? Or a delicious salmon salad for lunch?

Don't be afraid of fat - your brain is about 60% fat, after all! The right fats can help reduce inflammation, support neurotransmitter function, and even aid in the absorption of nutrients from other foods.

Feeling sharper already? That's your brain saying thank you for the premium fuel!

Day 6: Antioxidant Adventure
We're in the home stretch now! Today we're focusing on antioxidants - your body's defense against oxidative stress, which can wreak havoc on both your gut and your brain.

Berries, dark leafy greens, dark chocolate (yes, really!), and green tea are all packed with antioxidants. How about a spinach and blueberry smoothie to start your day? Or a square of dark chocolate as an afternoon pick-me-up?

Remember, variety is key. Different colors in fruits and vegetables indicate different types of antioxidants, so aim for a rainbow on your plate.

By now, you might be noticing clearer skin, better digestion, and improved mood. Your gut and brain are high-fiving each other!

Day 7: Mindful Meals

It's the final day of our gut reboot, and we're bringing it all together. Today is about mindful eating, paying attention to what, when, and how you eat.

Start your day with a moment of gratitude for your food. Chew slowly, savoring each bite. Put your fork down between mouthfuls. These simple practices can dramatically improve digestion and help you tune into your body's hunger and fullness cues.

Today's also about reflecting on the past week. What changes have you noticed? How do you feel compared to day one? Maybe keep a journal to track your progress.

Remember, this isn't about perfection. It's about progress and creating sustainable habits. Maybe you've discovered new foods you love, or perhaps you've noticed how certain foods make you feel. These insights are gold for your ongoing gut-brain health journey.

Congratulations! You've completed the 7-day gut reboot. But remember, this is just the beginning. Your gut and brain are in a constant conversation, and now you have the tools to keep that conversation positive and productive.

Moving forward, aim to incorporate elements from each day into your regular routine. Experiment, find your perfect combination. Your gut is as unique as you are, so listen to your body and adjust accordingly.

First Week Transformation: What to Expect (Spoiler: It's Awesome)

Day 1-2: The Gut Reset Rollercoaster

Buckle up, buttercup! The first couple days might feel like you're on a wild ride at the stomach-brain amusement park. Your body's likely throwing a little tantrum as you ditch the junk and introduce cleaner eats. Don't freak out if you're feeling a bit off – it's totally normal.

You might experience:

• Slight headaches (your brain's sugar withdrawal drama)

• Mild fatigue (your body's adjusting, like a computer rebooting)

• Occasional stomach gurgles (your gut bacteria are having a block party)

Pro tip: Stay hydrated! Water's your new BFF. It'll help flush out toxins and keep things moving smoothly.

Day 3-4: The Fog Starts to Lift

By now, you're probably thinking, "Hey, this isn't so bad!" That's the spirit! Your body's starting to get with the program, and you might notice some pretty cool changes:

• Mental clarity creeping in (like wiping a foggy mirror)

• Improved mood (random smiles? Yep, that's normal)

• Better sleep quality (hello, sweet dreams!)

Here's the deal: your gut bacteria are adapting to their new, healthier menu. They're multiplying faster than gossip at a high school reunion, and the good guys are finally outnumbering the troublemakers.

Fun fact: Did you know your gut produces about 95% of your body's serotonin? That's right, the happy hormone! So when your gut's doing better, your mood follows suit. It's like your belly's throwing a happiness party and your brain scored a VIP invite.

Day 5-6: Energy Surge and Craving Control

Hold onto your hats, folks, because things are about to get interesting! Around day 5 or 6, many people experience what I like to call the "gut-brain awakening." It's like your body suddenly remembers how awesome it feels to be healthy.

What's in store:
• Increased energy (without the caffeine jitters)
• Reduced cravings (bye-bye, 3 PM vending machine raids)
• Clearer skin (hello, natural glow!)

Let's talk cravings for a sec. You know that voice in your head that usually screams for cookies at midnight? It might start to pipe down. Why? Your blood sugar's stabilizing, and your gut bacteria are no longer demanding junk food like hangry toddlers.

Remember Jessica, a reader who tried this program? She said, "By day 6, I realized I hadn't thought about chocolate in 24 hours. That's a miracle for this former chocoholic!"

Day 7: The "A-ha!" Moment

Welcome to day 7, champ! This is often when people have their big "a-ha!" moment. Suddenly, the connection between your gut and your mind isn't just some woo-woo theory, it's your new reality.

What you might experience:
• Significantly improved mood stability
• Enhanced focus and concentration
• A general sense of well-being (like a mental hug)

One participant, Mike, described it like this: "It was like someone turned up the volume on life. Colors seemed brighter, my thoughts clearer. I hadn't realized how 'meh' I felt before until I experienced this change."

The Science Behind Your Transformation

Now, I know what you're thinking. "This sounds too good to be true!" But there's solid scientific foundation backing up your remarkable transformation.

1. Inflammation Reduction: By eliminating inflammatory foods, you're basically putting out the fire in your gut. Less inflammation means better nutrient absorption and improved communication between your gut and brain.

2. Microbiome Diversity: Your new diet is like sending reinforcements to the good bacteria in your gut. A diverse microbiome is linked to better mental health, improved immune function, and even weight management.

3. Neurotransmitter Production: Remember that serotonin fun fact? Your gut is working overtime to produce mood-regulating neurotransmitters, helping stabilize your emotions and improve your overall sense of well-being.

4. Vagus Nerve Activation: This superhighway between your gut and brain is humming with positive messages, improving your stress response and emotional regulation.

Dealing with Detox Symptoms

Now, let's keep it real. While many people feel fantastic by week's end, some might experience mild detox symptoms. This is your body's way of clearing out the gunk. Common symptoms include:

• Mild headaches
• Temporary fatigue
• Slight digestive upset

Don't worry, these are usually short-lived. Think of it as your body's spring cleaning – a little messy at first, but so worth it in the end.

Tips for Maximizing Your First Week:
1. Journal your experience. Noting changes in mood, energy, and physical sensations can be incredibly motivating.

2. Get moving. Gentle exercise like yoga or walking can aid digestion and boost your mood.

3. Prioritize sleep. Your body's doing important repair work while you snooze.

4. Stay social. Share your journey with friends or join our online community for support.

5. Practice mindfulness. Taking a few minutes each day to check in with yourself can enhance the gut-brain connection.

What's Next?

As amazing as this first week is, it's just the beginning. Your gut-brain axis will continue to strengthen, leading to long-term improvements in your mental and physical health.

In the coming weeks, you might notice:

• Even stable moods and emotions

• Improved stress resilience

• Better cognitive function

• Potential improvements in chronic health conditions

Remember, everyone's journey is unique. Some people feel like new humans after just a few days, while for others, the changes are more subtle. The key is patience and consistency.

As we wrap up this chapter, I want you to take a moment to celebrate your progress. You've taken a huge step towards transforming your health, and that's no small feat. Get ready for an exciting journey ahead.

Eating for Your Emotions: Menus to Beat the Blues and Calm the Crazies

Let's face it – we've all been there. One minute you're fine, the next you're diving headfirst into a pint of ice cream, wondering where it all went wrong. But what if I told you that your gut might be the puppet master pulling your emotional strings? Buckle up, because we're about to embark on a wild ride through the tasty world of mood-boosting meals.

The Emotional Eating Rollercoaster

Remember that time you inhaled an entire pizza after a brutal breakup? Or when you stress-ate your way through a bag of chips before a big presentation? Turns out, your gut was probably egging you on like a mischievous little gremlin. But here's the kicker – we can flip the script and use food to our advantage.

The Gut-Mood Connection: It's Not Just in Your Head
Your gut isn't just a food processor – it's a bustling metropolis of bacteria that have a direct line to your brain. These tiny tenants are constantly chattering away, influencing everything from your cravings to your mental state. So when we talk about "gut feelings," we're not just spouting poetic nonsense.

Mood Food 101: Your Edible Emotional Toolkit

Ready to eat your way to a better mood? Let's break down some all-star ingredients that'll have you feeling groovy in no time:

1. The Serotonin Superstars:
   - Turkey: Not just for Thanksgiving food comas anymore! This bird is packed with tryptophan, a precursor to serotonin.

- Eggs: The incredible, edible mood-lifter. Rich in protein and B vitamins, they're like little ovals of happiness.

- Cheese: Who knew your late-night quesadilla habit could be therapeutic? Dairy products are tryptophan powerhouses.

2. The Omega-3 Dream Team:

- Fatty fish: Salmon, mackerel, and sardines are like edible antidepressants.

- Walnuts: These brainy-looking nuts are brain food, quite literally.

- Flaxseeds: Tiny but mighty, these seeds pack an omega-3 punch.

3. The Probiotic Party:

- Yogurt: A creamy dose of good bacteria to keep your gut gremlins in check.

- Kimchi: Spice up your life (and your gut) with this Korean fermented cabbage.

- Kombucha: The fizzy, funky drink that's like a spa day for your insides.

4. The Magnesium Magicians:

- Dark chocolate: Finally, an excuse to indulge! Dark chocolate is rich in magnesium, a natural relaxant.

- Avocados: Nature's butter is also a mood-smoothing superstar.

- Spinach: Popeye was onto something – this leafy green is a magnesium goldmine.

Crafting Your Mood-Boosting Menu

Now that we've got our ingredient list, let's whip up some meals that'll have your taste buds doing the happy dance and your brain singing your praises.

Breakfast: The "Morning magic" Power Bowl

Mix Greek yogurt with a handful of walnuts, a sprinkle of flaxseeds, and a drizzle of honey. Top with sliced banana and a square of dark chocolate. It's like a hug for your gut and a high-five for your brain.

Lunch: The "No More Midday Slump" Salad

Toss spinach leaves with grilled salmon, sliced avocado, and a handful of cherry tomatoes. Dress with a lemon-olive oil vinaigrette and sprinkle with pumpkin seeds. This powerhouse will keep you energized and focused all afternoon.

Dinner: The "Comfort Food Without the Guilt" Plate

Roast a turkey breast and serve it alongside a scoop of kimchi and some steamed broccoli. Add a small baked sweet potato for some complex carbs. It's like Thanksgiving dinner's cooler, mood-boosting cousin.

Snack Attack: The "3 PM Slump Buster"

Whip up a quick smoothie with kefir, frozen berries, a handful of spinach, and a tablespoon of cocoa powder. It's probiotic-rich, antioxidant-packed, and just sweet enough to curb those cookie cravings.

The "Netflix and Chill" Platter

For those nights when you're tempted to eat your feelings, prep a tray with sliced turkey, cubes of cheese, whole grain crackers, and a handful of walnuts. Add some dark chocolate-covered almonds for a sweet finish. It's indulgent enough to feel like a treat, but balanced enough to keep your mood stable.

Beyond the Plate: Mindful Munchies

Remember, the art of eating is just as important as the food itself. Here are some tips to maximize your mood-boosting meals:

1. Slow down, speedracer: Chew thoroughly and savor each bite. Your gut and brain need time to communicate.
2. Ditch the distractions: Turn off the TV and put away your phone. Mindful eating helps you tune into your body's signals.
3. Hydrate, hydrate, hydrate: Sometimes thirst masquerades as hunger or moodiness. Keep that water bottle handy!
4. Eat the rainbow: A diverse diet means a diverse gut microbiome, which translates to a happier you.
5. Plan ahead: Meal prep when you're in a good mood to set yourself up for success during stressful times.

The Emotional Eating Emergency Kit

Life happens, and sometimes you need a quick mood fix. Keep these essential items for emotional eating crises;

- Dark chocolate-covered almonds: For when you need a sweet hit of magnesium and healthy fats.

- Individual packets of nut butter: Protein and healthy fats in a convenient, portion-controlled package.

- Herbal tea bags: Sometimes the ritual of brewing tea is as soothing as the drink itself.

- Single-serve Greek yogurt: A protein-packed snack that's also rich in probiotics.

- Roasted seaweed snacks: A low-calorie, mineral-rich alternative to chips.

Remember, food is powerful, but it's not a cure-all. If you're struggling with persistent mood issues, don't hesitate to reach out to a healthcare professional.

In conclusion, eating for your emotions isn't about drowning your sorrows in a tub of cookie dough (tempting as that may be). It's about nourishing your body and your mind with foods that support your emotional well-being. By choosing mood-boosting ingredients and crafting balanced meals, you're not just feeding your belly, you're feeding your happiness. So the next time you're tempted to stress-eat your way through the pantry, remember: your next meal could be the difference between riding the emotional rollercoaster and finding your zen. Choose wisely, eat joyfully, and watch your mood soar!

5-Minute Fixes: Quick Ways to Boost Your Gut-Brain Health

Let's face it – we're all busy. Between work, family, and trying to squeeze in a social life, who has time for hour-long meditation sessions or elaborate meal prep? But here's the thing: your gut-brain connection doesn't care about your packed schedule. It needs love, and it needs it now.

Good news, though! You don't need to overhaul your entire life to start feeling better. These lightning-fast tricks will give your gut and brain a boost, even when you're short on time.

1. The Two-Minute Tummy Massage

Feeling stressed? Your gut probably is too. Try this: Place your hands on your belly, right below your rib cage. Using gentle pressure, move your hands in a circular motion, clockwise (the direction your colon moves). Do this for two minutes while taking slow, deep breaths. This simple massage can help stimulate digestion, release tension, and kick-start your gut's feel-good signals to your brain.

2. kickstart Your Life (and Your Metabolism)

Next time you're in the kitchen, reach for the cinnamon. A quick dash on your morning coffee or oatmeal isn't just tasty – it's like a wake-up call for your metabolism. Cinnamon has been shown to help balance blood sugar, which can reduce cravings and mood swings. Plus, its antimicrobial properties give your gut flora a helping hand.

3. The 60-Second Squat

Sitting all day is a gut-health nightmare. Take a minute – literally – to do some squats. They engage your core, get things moving in your intestines, and release endorphins.

Aim for 15-20 squats, or as many as you can do in a minute. Bonus: your legs will thank you too!

4. Hydrate, But Make It Fancy

We all know we should drink more water, but plain H2O can get boring. Try this gut-loving twist: Fill a large glass with water, add a slice of lemon (great for digestion), a few mint leaves (calms the stomach), and a small pinch of sea salt (helps with mineral absorption). This spa-worthy drink takes seconds to prepare and sips like a treat while hydrating your gut and brain.

5. The Gratitude Gut-Check

This one's for your brain and belly. Take 30 seconds to jot down three things you're grateful for. Focusing on gratitude has been shown to reduce stress hormones like cortisol, which wreak havoc on your gut. Less stress means a happier digestive system, which in turn sends more positive signals to your brain. It's a beautiful cycle, and it starts with just half a minute of appreciation.

6. Probiotic Power-Up

Keep a quality probiotic supplement by your toothbrush. Pop one each morning as part of your routine. This daily dose of good bacteria can help balance your gut microbiome over time, leading to improved digestion and even better mood regulation.

7. The Breath of Fire

This yogic breathing technique is like an espresso shot for your gut-brain axis. Sit comfortably and take a few normal breaths. Then, start exhaling forcefully through your nose, followed by a passive inhale. Do this at a rate of about one breath per second for 30 seconds. This energizing breath stimulates your digestive fire, wakes up your brain, and can even help with bloating.

8. Green Tea Time-Out

Swap one of your daily coffees for green tea. It's packed with L-theanine, an amino acid that promotes relaxation without drowsiness. This calm-but-alert state is ideal for gut health, reducing stress-related digestive issues. Plus, green tea's antioxidants are like a cleanup crew for your insides.

9. The 3-3-3 Grounding Technique

Feeling anxious? This quick mindfulness exercise can help settle both your mind and your stomach. Name three things you can see, three things you can hear, and three things you can feel. This simple act of grounding yourself in the present moment can interrupt the stress response that plays havoc with your digestion.

10. Sole Searching

No, not the emotional kind – we're talking about sole water. Mix a teaspoon of high-quality Himalayan salt in a glass of water before bed. In the morning, add a teaspoon of this salt solution to your first glass of water. This mineral-rich drink can help stimulate digestion, balance pH levels, and support your body's natural detox processes.

11. Laugh It Up

Pull up a funny video or call that friend who always cracks you up. A good belly laugh isn't just fun – it's medicine for your gut-brain axis. Laughter reduces stress hormones, increases feel-good endorphins, and can even boost your immune system. Plus, the physical act of laughing gives your abs and diaphragm a mini-workout, aiding digestion.

12. Oil Pulling Surprise

This Ayurvedic practice isn't just for oral health. Swish a tablespoon of coconut oil in your mouth for 5 minutes while you're getting ready in the morning. It may help pull toxins from your body, reduce inflammation, and even improve gut health by reducing the overall bacterial load in your system.

13. The Gut-Love Playlist

Create a 5-minute playlist of songs that make you feel amazing. Music has been shown to reduce cortisol levels and increase dopamine – a double win for your gut-brain connection. Dance it out for an extra mood and digestion boost!

14. Sunlight Snack Break

Step outside for a 5-minute sunlight snack. The vitamin D boost supports both gut health and mood regulation. Plus, the act of mindfully eating in natural light can help reset your circadian rhythms, which play a crucial role in digestion and mental health.

15. Tongue Scraping Ritual

This might sound weird, but hear me out. Tongue scraping is an ancient practice that's making a comeback. A quick scrape in the morning can remove toxins and bacteria that accumulated overnight, preventing them from being reabsorbed. Less toxins mean a happier gut and a clearer mind.

Remember, the key to these 5-minute fixes is consistency. You don't have to do them all every day – pick a few that resonate with you and make them part of your routine. Your gut and your brain will thank you, and you might just find yourself with more energy, better moods, and a happier belly.

Now, who said taking care of your gut-brain axis had to be time-consuming? With these quick tricks up your sleeve, you're well on your way to a healthier, happier you – five minutes at a time.

Chapter 3: Food Is Your New Chill Pill

Eating Your Way to Mental Wellness

Envision You're stressed out, anxious, maybe even a bit down in the dumps. What's your go-to solution? For many of us, it's reaching for that pint of ice cream or bag of chips. But what if I told you that food could actually be the key to unlocking your inner zen – and not in the way you might think?

Welcome to the revolutionary world of nutritional psychiatry, where your plate becomes a powerful tool for mental health. It's time to ditch the idea that food is just fuel or comfort. Instead, let's explore how it can be your secret weapon in the battle against stress, anxiety, and even depression.

The Mood Food Revolution

Remember when your grandma said, "You are what you eat"? Well, she was onto something big. Scientists are now discovering that the connection between our gut and our brain is so strong, it's like they're best friends who text each other 24/7. This gut-brain axis is reshaping how we think about mental health, and it all starts with what's on your fork.

But here's the kicker – we're not talking about bland, boring "health food" that tastes like cardboard. Nope, we're diving into a world of delicious eats that not only tantalize your taste buds but also give your brain a big, warm hug. Think vibrant berries, rich dark chocolate, and even that morning cup of joe (yes, really!).

Serotonin: The Happiness Hormone Hiding in Your Kitchen

Let's talk about serotonin, often called the "happiness hormone." Did you know that about 95% of it is produced in your gut? That's right – your belly is basically a serotonin factory. And guess what influences this production? That's right – the food you consume.

Foods rich in tryptophan, like turkey, eggs, and cheese, are serotonin superstars. But don't forget about complex carbs –

they help your body absorb tryptophan more effectively. So that sweet potato or whole grain bread isn't just delicious; it's also helping your brain chill out.

The Omega-3 Connection: Fish for Your Feelings

Ever heard the phrase "brain food"? Well, when it comes to omega-3 fatty acids, it's spot on. These little nutrient powerhouses are like premium fuel for your noggin. Found in fatty fish like salmon, mackerel, and sardines, omega-3s help build brain cells and reduce inflammation – a big culprit in mood disorders.

But what if you're not a fish fan? No worries! Walnuts, flaxseeds, and chia seeds are plant-based omega-3 rockstars. Sprinkle them on your morning yogurt or toss them in a salad for a brain-boosting crunch.

Probiotic Paradise: Feeding Your Inner Ecosystem

Now, let's dive into the wild world of probiotics. These friendly bacteria are like tiny gardeners for your gut, cultivating a healthy microbiome. And a happy gut microbiome means a happier you.

Fermented foods are your ticket to probiotic paradise. We're talking tangy yogurt, zippy kimchi, and fizzy kombucha. Each spoonful or sip is like sending a peace treaty to the war zone in your belly, calming inflammation and boosting those feel-good chemicals.

But don't stop at probiotics – say hello to prebiotics too. These are the foods that feed your good gut bacteria. Think garlic, onions, and bananas. It's like laying out a welcome mat for the good guys in your gut.

The Sweet Truth About Dark Chocolate

Here's some news that'll make you smile: dark chocolate is a legitimate mood-booster. It's packed with compounds that increase serotonin production and reduce the stress hormone cortisol. Plus, it just feels indulgent, doesn't it? Opt for chocolate with at least 70% cocoa for maximum benefits (and minimum guilt).

Spice Up Your Life (and Your Mood)

Turmeric, the golden spice of Indian cuisine, is more than just a pretty face. Its active compound, curcumin, has powerful anti-inflammatory properties that may help alleviate symptoms of depression. Sprinkle it in your smoothies, add it to roasted veggies, or sip on a warming turmeric latte for a cozy mood lift.

And let's not forget about saffron, the world's most expensive spice. Studies have shown it can be as effective as some antidepressants in treating mild to moderate depression. A little goes a long way, so add a pinch to your rice dishes or steep it in tea for a luxurious mood-enhancing treat.

The Magic of Mindful Eating

Now, it's not just about what you eat, but how you eat it. Mindful eating – paying full attention to your food without distractions – can transform your relationship with meals and boost your mood in the process. It's like meditation, but with the added bonus of delicious flavors.

Try this: Next time you eat, put away your phone, turn off the TV, and really focus on your food. Notice the colors, textures, and aromas. Chew slowly and savor each bite. This practice not only enhances your enjoyment of food but also helps reduce stress and emotional eating.

Crafting Your Mood-Boosting Menu

So, how do you apply this practically? Start by building your meals around a rainbow of fruits and vegetables. These plant powerhouses are packed with vitamins, minerals, and antioxidants that support brain health. Aim for at least five different colors on your plate each day.

Don't forget your proteins – they're crucial for neurotransmitter production. Lean meats, fish, beans, and lentils are all great options. And include healthy fats like avocados, olive oil, and nuts to keep your brain cells firing on all cylinders.

Hydration Station: The Overlooked Mood Booster

Here's a simple yet often overlooked mood hack: drink more water. Dehydration can masquerade as fatigue, irritability, and even mild depression. Keep a water bottle handy and jazz it up with slices of lemon, cucumber, or a sprig of mint for a refreshing mood lift.

The Coffee Conundrum: Friend or Foe?

Let's address the elephant in the room – coffee. For years, we've been told it's bad for us, but recent research suggests moderate coffee consumption can actually boost mood and cognitive function. The key is moderation – aim for no more than 3-4 cups a day and cut off the caffeine by early afternoon to avoid sleep disruptions.

Creating Your Personal Food-Mood Journal

Everyone's gut is unique, so what works for one person might not work for another. That's where a food-mood journal comes in handy. For a few weeks, jot down what you eat and how you feel afterward. Look for patterns – maybe you notice you feel energized after your morning smoothie but sluggish after a heavy pasta lunch. This personal data is gold for crafting your ideal mood-boosting menu.

The Social Aspect of Eating

The act of sharing a meal with loved ones can have a profound impact on your well being. Social connection is a huge mood booster, and combining it with nourishing food is a double whammy for your mental health. Plan regular dinner dates with friends or family cook-offs for a hearty dose of laughter and love alongside your nutrients.

Navigating the Grocery Store for Brain Health

Armed with all this knowledge, your next trip to the grocery store might feel a bit overwhelming. Here's a pro tip: stick to the perimeter of the store. That's where you'll find the fresh produce, lean proteins, and dairy products. The inner aisles are often filled with processed foods that can wreak havoc on your gut-brain axis.

When you do venture into the center aisles, become a label detective. Look for foods with short ingredient lists full of words you can pronounce. Your gut (and your brain) will thank you.

The Power of Meal Prep

Setting yourself up for success is key when it comes to mood-boosting eating. Allocate a few hours each week to meal prep. Chop veggies, cook grains, and prepare proteins in advance. This way, when stress hits and you're tempted to reach for junk food, you'll have healthy options ready to go.

Embracing the Journey

Remember, transforming your diet isn't about perfection – it's about progress. There will be days when you indulge in comfort foods, and that's okay. The goal is to gradually shift towards a way of eating that nourishes both your body and your mind.

As you embark on this food-as-medicine journey, be patient with yourself. It might take a few weeks to notice significant changes in your mood. But stick with it – the results can be truly life-changing.

In conclusion, your kitchen is now your pharmacy, and your fork is your new prescription pad. By harnessing the power of nutrient-dense, gut-friendly foods, you're not just eating, you're actively participating in your mental health care. So the next time stress, anxiety, or the blues come knocking, don't just reach for any old snack. Reach for foods that feed your happiness, calm your nerves, and brighten your outlook. Your gut, your brain, and your taste buds will all be singing your praises.

Eat Your Way to Happy: Brain-Boosting Superfoods

Ever caught yourself reaching for that pint of ice cream after a rough day? Or maybe you've noticed how a greasy burger seems to slow your thoughts to a crawl? Well, buckle up, buttercup, because we're about to embark on a wild ride through your kitchen that'll revolutionize your mental health.

Picture you're standing in front of your fridge, and instead of seeing boring old vegetables, you're looking at an arsenal of mood-boosting, brain-fog-busting superheroes. Sounds too good to be true? Stick with me, and I'll show you how to transform your grocery list into a prescription for happiness.

The Mood-Food Connection: More Than Just Comfort Eating

We've all heard the phrase "you are what you eat," but let's kick it up a notch. You think what you eat. Your brain, that magnificent blob of gray matter, is constantly chattering with your gut, and what you feed that gut can make or break your mental state.

Think of your gut as a picky toddler. Feed it junk, and it'll throw a tantrum that your brain can't ignore. But nourish it with the right stuff, and it'll sing a happy song that has your neurons dancing with joy.

Superfoods: Your Gut's New BFFs
Now, let's meet the all-star lineup of brain-boosting superfoods that'll have your gut and brain high-fiving each other:

1. Blueberries: The Tiny Blue Defenders
   These little blue dynamos are like bouncers for your brain, fighting off the rowdy free radicals that try to crash the party in your head. Packed with antioxidants, they help keep your neural pathways clear, so your thoughts can zoom along like a bullet train.

2. Fatty Fish: The Omega-3 Omega

Salmon, mackerel, and sardines are swimming in omega-3 fatty acids, the building blocks of happy brain cells. Think of these fish as the construction workers of your mental skyscraper, constantly repairing and upgrading your brain's infrastructure.

3. Dark Chocolate: The Sweet Savior

Yes, you read that right. Dark chocolate (the darker, the better) is packed with flavonoids that increase blood flow to the brain. It's like giving your brain a spa day, complete with improved mood and sharper focus. Just don't go overboard – moderation is key, unless you want a sugar crash to rain on your brain parade.

4. Fermented Foods: The Gut's Glee Club

Kimchi, sauerkraut, and kefir might sound like the punchline to a food joke, but they're serious business for your gut health. These probiotic powerhouses introduce good bacteria to your gut, creating a harmonious microbiome that sings sweet nothings to your brain.

5. Leafy Greens: The Crispy Cleansers

Spinach, kale, and their leafy friends are like a detox spa for your brain. Rich in folate and other B vitamins, they help produce mood-regulating neurotransmitters. So next time you're feeling down, try a big ol' salad instead of drowning your sorrows in a bag of chips.

6. Nuts and Seeds: The Crunchy Mood Lifters

Walnuts, almonds, pumpkin seeds – these little nuggets of joy are packed with zinc, magnesium, and healthy fats. They're like nature's chill pills, helping to ease anxiety and boost your overall mood. Plus, the satisfying crunch is a bonus for stress relief.

7. Turmeric: The Golden Gladiator

This vibrant spice isn't just for curry. Curcumin, the active compound in turmeric, is a fierce warrior against inflammation and oxidative stress. It's like sending a squadron of tiny yellow superheroes to defend your brain's honor.

Putting It All Together: Your Brain's Gourmet Feast

Now, I know what you're thinking. "Great, I've got a list of superfoods. Now what?" Fear not, my hungry friend. Let's whip up a day of delicious, brain-boosting meals that'll have your neurons doing the happy dance.

Breakfast: Berry Blue Brain Boost Bowl

Start your day with a bang by blending up a smoothie bowl. Mix blueberries, spinach, and a dollop of Greek yogurt for probiotics. Top it with a sprinkle of walnuts and pumpkin seeds for that perfect crunch. Your brain will be so jazzed, it might just solve world peace before lunch.

Lunch: The Omega Upgrade Salad

Toss together a vibrant salad with leafy greens, chunks of grilled salmon, and a rainbow of veggies. Drizzle it with an olive oil and turmeric dressing for an extra brain boost. It's like sending your neurons to a five-star resort for lunch.

Dinner: Fermented Feast

Grill up some mackerel and serve it alongside a heap of kimchi or sauerkraut. Add a side of roasted vegetables sprinkled with turmeric for good measure. Your gut bacteria will be throwing a party, and your brain will be the guest of honor.

Dessert: Dark Delight

Cap off your day with a small square of dark chocolate. Savor it slowly, and feel those flavonoids work their magic. It's the perfect nightcap for your brain.

The Proof is in the Pudding (The Sugar-Free, Brain-Boosting Pudding)

Now, I know this all sounds great in theory, but you're probably wondering, "Does this stuff really work?" Well, let me tell you a story about my friend Jake. Jake used to be a stress ball with legs. His idea of a balanced diet was making sure he had a burger in both hands.

After I nagged him into trying this brain-food approach for a month, the change was like night and day. Not only did he have more energy, but his mood stabilized, and he swore his thinking was clearer than it had been in years. He went from grumpy cat to motivational poster child in weeks.

But don't just take my word for it. A study published in the "American Journal of Clinical Nutrition" found that people who followed a diet rich in these brain-boosting foods showed improved cognitive function and a decreased risk of depression. It's like these foods are little edible therapists, working round the clock to keep your mental health in check.

The Challenge: Your Brain's 30-Day Makeover
Here's where the rubber meets the road, folks. I challenge you to a 30-day brain-food makeover. Incorporate these superfoods into your daily diet and keep a mood journal. Track your energy levels, your ability to focus, and your overall sense of well-being.

I bet you a virtual high-five that by the end of those 30 days, you'll be feeling like a new person. Your gut will be singing your praises, and your brain? Well, it might just send you a thank-you note.

Remember, transforming your mental health through nutrition isn't about perfection. It's about progress. So if you slip up and face-plant into a pizza one night, don't sweat it. Just get back on track with your next meal. Your brain is in this for the long haul, and so are you.

In conclusion, eating your way to happiness isn't just a catchy phrase – it's a delicious reality. By fueling your body with these brain-boosting superfoods, you're not just satisfying your hunger; you're feeding your future. A future where your gut and brain work in perfect harmony, and where mental clarity and emotional stability are on the menu every single day.

So, are you ready to eat your way to a happier, healthier you? Your brain is waiting, fork in hand. Let's dig in!

Nature's Prozac: The Serotonin Secret Hiding in Your Fridge

You're standing in front of your open fridge, hunting for a snack to lift your spirits. Little do you know, the answer to your mood woes might be right there, nestled between the wilting lettuce and last night's leftovers. Welcome to the wild world of serotonin-boosting foods – nature's very own antidepressants!

Now, before you roll your eyes and reach for that pint of ice cream, hear me out. We're about to embark on a culinary adventure that could revolutionize the way you think about food and mood. Buckle up, buttercup – it's time to turn your kitchen into a happiness laboratory!

The Serotonin Saga: More Than Just a Brain Chemical

Let's begin with a dose of science, shall we? Serotonin, often dubbed the "happy hormone," is like the VIP bouncer at the hottest club in your brain. It's calling the shots on your mood, sleep, appetite, and even how well you handle stress. But here's the kicker – a whopping 95% of your body's serotonin is actually produced in your gut. Mind-blowing, right?

This gut-brain tango is more intricate than a Strictly Come Dancing routine. Your belly bugs (aka gut microbiome) are the unsung heroes in this production, playing a crucial role in serotonin synthesis. So, when we talk about eating for happiness, we're not just feeding our taste buds – we're catering to an entire microscopic civilization in our intestines!

The Tryptophan Train: All Aboard for Bliss Ville

let's get down to the nitty-gritty. Serotonin production starts with an amino acid called tryptophan. Think of tryptophan as the VIP guest that needs to be escorted into the exclusive serotonin nightclub. But here's the rub – your body can't produce tryptophan on its own. It's like trying to get into a fancy party without an invitation. The solution? You've got to sneak it in through your diet!

Foods rich in tryptophan are your golden ticket to Bliss Ville. We're talking about:

1. Turkey: Not just for Thanksgiving food comas anymore!

2. Eggs: The incredible, edible mood-lifters.

3. Cheese: Finally, a reason to justify that midnight cheddar binge.

4. Nuts and seeds: Especially pumpkin seeds – who knew these little guys packed such a punch?

5. Salmon: Swimming upstream to Happiness Harbor.

But wait, there's a plot twist! Tryptophan is a bit of a diva and needs some backup dancers to really shine. Enter carbohydrates – the unsung heroes in this serotonin soap opera.

Carbs: The Unsung Heroes of the Serotonin Saga

Carbs have gotten a bad rap lately, but in the world of serotonin, they're the real MVPs. Here's the deal: eating carbs triggers the release of insulin, which helps clear other amino acids from your bloodstream. This gives tryptophan a clear path to your brain, like a red carpet rolled out just for it.

But before you face-plant into a bowl of pasta, let's talk about the right kind of carbs. We're not talking about refined sugar or processed junk. Oh no, we're aiming for the wholesome stuff:

1. Sweet potatoes: Nature's candy with a side of mood boost.
2. Quinoa: The grain that thinks it's a superhero.
3. Oats: Not just for horses and health nuts anymore.
4. Bananas: The OG mood food (and conveniently shaped like a smile).

The key is to pair these carbs with your tryptophan-rich foods. It's like setting up your taste buds on a blind date with your neurotransmitters. Romantic, isn't it?

Fermentation Nation: Probiotic Power-Ups

Now, let's talk about fermented foods – the funky, tangy superheroes of the gut-brain axis. These probiotic powerhouses are like a support group for your gut bacteria, helping them flourish and, in turn, boosting serotonin production.

Some fermented favorites to add to your shopping list:

1. Kimchi: Korean cuisine's gift to your gut.
2. Kombucha: The fizzy drink that's actually good for you.
3. Kefir: Like yogurt, but with an attitude.
4. Sauerkraut: Not just for hot dogs anymore!

Incorporating these foods into your diet is like sending a care package to your gut microbiome. Happy gut bugs = happy you!

The Dark Horse: Chocolate's Mood-Boosting Magic

I know what you're thinking – "Finally, they're going to tell me chocolate is good for me!" Well, you're in luck, my cacao-craving friend. Dark chocolate (the darker, the better) isn't just delicious; it's a mood-boosting powerhouse.

Dark chocolate contains tryptophan, but it also has other tricks up its silky sleeve. It stimulates the production of endorphins, the brain's natural feel-good chemicals. Plus, it contains phenylethylamine, a compound that's been dubbed the "love drug" due to its ability to quicken your heartbeat and make you feel giddy – kind of like falling in love, but with less awkward first dates.

Aim for chocolate with at least 70% cocoa content. It's like sending your taste buds and your neurotransmitters on a luxurious spa day.

Liquid Sunshine: Hydration and Mood

Before you slam the fridge door shut, let's not forget about good old H2O. Dehydration can be a real mood-killer, leaving you feeling sluggish, irritable, and downright cranky. Proper hydration is crucial for every bodily function, including the production and regulation of serotonin.

Jazz up your water intake with some mood-boosting infusions:

1. Lemon and mint: A refreshing combo that screams "Good morning, serotonin!"
2. Cucumber and basil: Like a spa day in a glass.
3. Strawberry and rosemary: Fancy enough to make you feel like you've got your life together.

Remember, every time you hydrate, you're basically giving your gut-brain axis a standing ovation.

The Serotonin Shopping List: Your Fridge's New Best Friends

Alright, let's recap and create the ultimate serotonin-boosting shopping list. Next time you hit the grocery store, keep an eye out for these mood-food all-stars:

1. Proteins: Turkey, eggs, cheese, salmon, tofu
2. Complex Carbs: Sweet potatoes, quinoa, oats, brown rice
3. Fruits: Bananas, kiwis, pineapples, plums
4. Veggies: Spinach, broccoli, asparagus
5. Nuts and Seeds: Pumpkin seeds, almonds, cashews
6. Fermented Foods: Kimchi, kombucha, kefir, sauerkraut
7. Treats: Dark chocolate (70%+ cocoa)
8. Beverages: Water, green tea, chamomile tea

Remember, variety is the spice of life – and the key to a well-fed, happy gut microbiome!

Conclusion: Your Fridge, Your Pharmacy

As we close the door on this fridge full of knowledge, remember that your kitchen is more than just a place to store leftovers and hide from social obligations. It's a treasure trove of mood-boosting potential, a natural pharmacy stocked with serotonin-stimulating wonders.

By mindfully incorporating these foods into your diet, you're not just eating – you're conducting a symphony of neurotransmitters, orchestrating a masterpiece of mental well-being. It's like being the DJ at the hottest brain-gut rave in town!

So, the next time you're feeling down, don't just grab the nearest comfort food. Take a moment to consider what your gut-brain axis is really craving. Your mood, and your microbiome, will thank you.

Feed Your Inner Zoo: All About Pre- and Probiotics

For an instance you're standing in front of your fridge, wondering what to eat. But here's the twist – you're not just feeding yourself. You're feeding trillions of tiny guests living in your gut. That's the wild world of your inner zoo!

Let's get real for a second. When most of us think about bacteria, we imagine nasty germs that make us sick. But hold onto your kombucha, folks, because I'm about to blow your mind. Your gut is home to a bustling metropolis of beneficial bacteria that can make or break your mental health. And the best part? You get to play zookeeper.

Enter pre- and probiotics – the dynamic duo of gut health. Think of prebiotics as the gourmet chef preparing a five-star meal for your gut bacteria, while probiotics are the VIP guests ready to party in your intestines. Together, they're like the ultimate power couple, working in harmony to keep your gut-brain axis humming along smoothly.

But wait, what exactly are these microscopic marvels?

Probiotics: The Gut's A-List Celebrities

Probiotics are live bacteria and yeasts that are good for your overall wellbeing, especially your digestive system. They're the cool kids of the gut world, and trust me, you want them at your party. These beneficial bugs help keep the bad bacteria in check, sort of like bouncers at an exclusive club.

Now, you might be thinking, "Hold up, I thought bacteria were bad news!" Well, not these guys. Probiotics are the unsung heroes of your body, working tirelessly to:

1. Boost your immune system (bye-bye, sniffles!)
2. Improve digestion (sayonara, bloating!)
3. Enhance nutrient absorption (hello, energy!)
4. Produce feel-good neurotransmitters (take that, bad mood!)

But here's where it gets really interesting. Some strains of probiotics are like tiny psychiatrists for your gut. They've been shown to help alleviate symptoms of anxiety and depression. How's that for a mood boost?

Prebiotics: The Unsung Heroes

Now, let's talk about prebiotics. If probiotics are the rock stars, prebiotics are the roadies – not as glamorous, but absolutely crucial to the show. These are specialized plant fibers that act as food for the good bacteria in your gut.

Think of prebiotics as fertilizer for your internal garden. They help the good bacteria grow and thrive, creating a lush, diverse ecosystem in your gut. And let me tell you, when it comes to gut health, diversity is the spice of life!

Some top-notch prebiotic foods include:

1. Jerusalem artichokes (don't worry, I can't pronounce it either)
2. Chicory root (sounds fancy, tastes great)
3. Garlic (vampire protection is just a bonus)
4. Onions (your breath might suffer, but your gut will thank you)

5. Bananas (nature's perfect snack just got perfecter)

The Pre- and Probiotic Tango

Here's where the magic happens. When you combine prebiotics and probiotics, it's like throwing the ultimate gut party. The prebiotics roll out the red carpet, creating the perfect environment for the probiotic VIPs to thrive.

This dynamic duo can work wonders for your gut-brain axis. By fostering a healthy gut environment, they help reduce inflammation, balance neurotransmitter production, and strengthen the gut barrier. Translation? You might just find yourself feeling happier, calmer, and sharper than ever before.

But don't just take my word for it. Let's hear from Sarah, a 35-year-old marketing exec who struggled with anxiety and brain fog for years:

"I was skeptical at first," Sarah admits. "But after incorporating pre- and probiotic-rich foods into my diet for a month, I felt like a fog had lifted. My anxiety decreased, and I could finally focus at work without feeling like my brain was stuck in molasses."

The Pre- and Probiotic Shopping List
Ready to stock up on these gut-friendly goodies? Here's your cheat sheet:

Probiotic-Rich Foods:
1. Yogurt (but watch out for added sugars!)
2. Kefir (like yogurt's cool, tangy cousin)
3. Sauerkraut (not just for hot dogs anymore)
4. Kimchi (Korea's gift to your gut)
5. Kombucha (the hipster drink that actually lives up to the hype)

Prebiotic Powerhouses:
1. Asparagus (yes, it makes your pee smell funny, but your gut bugs love it)
2. Leeks (the onion's sophisticated sibling)
3. Apples (one a day keeps the bad bacteria away)
4. Flaxseeds (tiny seeds, big impact)

5. Oats (not just for breakfast anymore)

The Supplement Situation

I know what you're thinking. "Can't I just swallow a pill and call it a day?" Well, you could, but where's the fun in that? While probiotic supplements can be beneficial, especially if you're on antibiotics or have specific health concerns, nothing beats the real deal from food sources.

If you do opt for supplements, remember this: quality matters. Look for products with multiple strains of bacteria and a high CFU (colony-forming unit) count. And always, always check with your doctor before starting any new supplement regimen.

The Gut-Brain Axis: A Love Story

Here's the bottom line, folks. Your gut and your brain are in a long-distance relationship, and pre- and probiotics are like the ultimate couples therapist. By nurturing your gut microbiome, you're essentially sending a love letter to your brain.

A healthy gut microbiome can:

1. Reduce inflammation (the root of many mental health issues)

2. Produce neurotransmitters like serotonin (hello, happiness!)

3. Strengthen your gut barrier (keeping the bad stuff out and the good stuff in)

4. Improve nutrient absorption (feeding your brain the good stuff)

So, the next time you're feeling down, anxious, or just plain foggy, remember this: the solution might just be in your gut. By feeding your inner zoo with a diverse array of pre- and probiotic foods, you're not just improving your digestive health – you're giving your brain a fighting chance at happiness and clarity.

Keto, Paleo, Vegan: Finding Your Gut-Brain Diet Style

Let's face it, the world of diets is a jungle. Everywhere you turn, there's another guru telling you they've cracked the code to optimal health. But here's the kicker: when it comes to your gut-brain connection, one size definitely doesn't fit all. So, buckle up, buttercup – we're about to dive into the wild world of dietary approaches that might just revolutionize your mental health.

First things first: why does your diet style even matter for your noggin? Well, imagine your gut as a bustling city, and the food you eat as the supplies coming in. The right supplies keep everything humming along smoothly, while the wrong ones can lead to riots in the streets (hello, inflammation!). And guess what? Your brain is like the mayor of this gut city, feeling every single up and down.

Now, let's break down these dietary heavyweights:

Keto: The Fat-Fueled Brain Boost

What if you're at a party, and your brain cells are doing the conga line, powered by... fat? Yep, you heard that right. The ketogenic diet, with its high-fat, low-carb approach, can turn your body into a fat-burning machine. But it's not just about shedding pounds – it's about feeding your brain its favorite fuel.

Here's the deal: when you cut out the carbs, your body starts producing ketones. These little molecules are like rocket fuel for your brain cells. Many keto enthusiasts report feeling sharper, more focused, and even experiencing a lift in mood. It's like giving your brain a shot of espresso, minus the jitters.

But (there's always a but, isn't there?), keto isn't a walk in the park for everyone. Some folks experience the "keto flu" as their body adjusts, feeling like they've been hit by a truck made of bacon. And let's be real – saying goodbye to bread can feel like breaking up with your high school sweetheart. Tragic, but sometimes necessary.

Paleo: Channeling Your Inner Caveman (or Woman)
Imagine if your great-great-great (add about a thousand more "greats") grandparents popped by for dinner. What would they eat? That's the basic idea behind the Paleo diet. It's all about getting back to our roots – literally.

The Paleo approach focuses on whole foods that our ancestors might have hunted or gathered. We're talking lean meats, fish, fruits, veggies, nuts, and seeds. The theory? Our bodies haven't evolved much since the Stone Age, so why should our diets?

For your gut-brain axis, Paleo can be a game-changer. By cutting out processed foods and potential irritants like grains and dairy, many people find their digestion improves dramatically. And when your gut's happy, your brain throws a party.

But here's the rub – strict Paleo can be tough to maintain in our modern world. Try explaining to your date why you're sniffing suspiciously at the restaurant bread basket like it might contain smallpox. Plus, some critics argue that we've evolved more than Paleo fans give us credit for. (Spoiler alert: we have.)

Vegan: Plant-Powered Brain Power
Now, let's swing to the other end of the spectrum. Vegan diets have exploded in popularity, and not just among the tie-dye and tambourine crowd. More and more folks are discovering the benefits of going all-in on plants.

For your gut-brain connection, a vegan diet can be like hiring a cleanup crew for your insides. All those plant fibers act like tiny scrub brushes, keeping your gut lining healthy and happy. Plus, plants are packed with polyphenols – compounds that act like bouncers, kicking out inflammation and oxidative stress.

Many vegans report feeling lighter, more energetic, and mentally clearer. It's like upgrading your body's operating system to the latest version. But (you knew this was coming), vegan diets require some serious planning to avoid nutritional pitfalls. B12 deficiency is no joke, folks – it can leave you feeling like your brain's been replaced with cotton candy.

Finding Your Gut-Brain Soulmate

So, how do you choose? Well, here's a radical idea: listen to your gut. Literally. Your body is the world's most sophisticated feedback system. It's constantly sending you signals about what's working and what's not.

Try this: spend a week really tuning into how different foods make you feel. Not just in your stomach, but in your mood, energy levels, and mental clarity. Keep a food diary if you're feeling fancy. You would be mesmerized at what you discover.

Maybe you'll find that a modified keto approach, with a bit more veggie variety, lights up your brain like Times Square on New Year's Eve. Or perhaps a mostly plant-based diet with the occasional wild-caught salmon makes you feel like you could solve world peace before breakfast.

The key is to be flexible and curious. Your perfect gut-brain diet might be a mash-up that would make a nutritionist's head spin. And that's okay! We're all unique snowflakes, with gut microbiomes as individual as our fingerprints.

Remember, this isn't about being perfect, it's about progress. Maybe you start with "Meatless Mondays" and see how you feel. Or you could try a 30-day Paleo challenge and track your mood. The possibilities are as endless as your grandma's advice on how to find a life partner.

The Plot Twist: It's Not Just About the Food

Here's where things get really interesting. While what you eat is crucial, how you eat might be just as important for your gut-brain harmony.

Ever heard of mindful eating? It's not just for Zen masters and yoga instructors. Taking the time to really savor your food, chewing slowly and appreciating each bite, can work wonders for your digestion and, by extension, your mental state.

And let's not forget about meal timing. Intermittent fasting has been making waves in the health world, and for good reason. Giving your gut a break can promote cellular repair and reduce inflammation. It's like sending your internal organs to a spa day.

The Final Course

At the end of the day (or meal), finding your ideal gut-brain diet style is a journey, not a destination. It's about tuning in to your body's wisdom and being willing to experiment.

Remember, the goal isn't to find a diet that looks good on Instagram. It's about discovering a way of eating that makes you feel alive, alert, and ready to tackle whatever life throws your way – whether that's a big presentation at work or just remembering where you left your car keys.

So go forth and explore! You might just stumble upon a dietary approach so perfect for you, it feels like it was written in the stars. Or at least in your DNA.

Intermittent Fasting: Give Your Gut a Break, Boost Your Brain

Envision you're sitting at your desk, clock ticking towards lunchtime, and your stomach starts its usual grumbling orchestra. But instead of reaching for that sandwich, you take a sip of water and carry on with your day. Sounds crazy, right?

Well, that's intermittent fasting for you, the eating pattern that's turning everything we thought we knew about nutrition on its head.

Now, before you roll your eyes and mutter "Here comes another fad diet," hear me out. Intermittent fasting isn't about menu, it's about schedule. It's like hitting the reset button on your body's internal systems, giving your hardworking gut a well-deserved vacation, and in turn, supercharging your brain.

The Gut-Brain Time-Share

Think of your body as a bustling city. Your gut is like the sanitation department, constantly processing and dealing with whatever you throw at it. Your brain? It's the city hall, making all the big decisions. Now, imagine if the sanitation department went on strike. City hall would have to divert resources to deal with the mess, right? That's essentially what happens when we eat all day long – our gut is always on duty, leaving less energy for our brain to do its thing.

Enter intermittent fasting. By creating designated periods of fasting, we're essentially giving our gut a chance to clock out, put its feet up, and binge-watch some cellular repair shows. And guess what? When your gut's on break, your brain gets to party.

The Cellular Cleanup Crew

During fasting periods, your body kicks into a process called autophagy. Fancy word, I know, but stick with me. Autophagy is like your body's own Marie Kondo – it goes through your cells, tidying up, getting rid of the junk, and keeping only what sparks joy (or in this case, what's necessary for optimal function).

This cellular spring cleaning is a big deal for your brain. It helps clear out damaged proteins that can lead to neurodegenerative diseases. It's like decluttering your mental attic, making space for clearer thinking, better memory, and improved focus. Who knew skipping breakfast could be so powerful?

The Gut's Second Wind

But let's not forget about our hardworking friend, the gut. Intermittent fasting gives it a chance to repair and regenerate.

It's like closing down a busy restaurant for renovations — when it reopens, everything runs more smoothly.

During fasting periods, the gut lining gets a chance to heal. This can lead to reduced inflammation, better nutrient absorption, and a happier, more diverse microbiome. And remember, a happy gut means a happy brain. They're like an old married couple – when one's thriving, the other can't help but perk up too.

The Neurotransmitter Boost

Now, let's talk brain chemicals. Intermittent fasting has been proven to increase protein production called brain-derived neurotrophic factor (BDNF). I know, another fancy term, but this one's worth remembering. BDNF works like a Miracle-Gro for your brain cells. It helps create new neurons and strengthens existing ones. More BDNF means better learning, improved memory, and even elevated mood. It's like giving your brain a superhero cape.

But that's not all. Fasting also triggers the release of norepinephrine, a neurotransmitter that helps with focus and attention. So, not only are you growing new brain cells, but you're also teaching the existing ones to pay better attention. It's a cognitive double whammy!

The Insulin Connection

Here's where things get really interesting. Intermittent fasting can help regulate insulin levels. Now, you would be thinking, "Isn't insulin solely about blood sugar? What's that got to do with my brain?" Well, buckle up, because we're about to connect some dots.

Insulin doesn't just manage blood sugar; it also plays a role in brain function. When insulin levels are constantly high (like when we're eating all day), it can lead to insulin resistance. And insulin resistance in the brain? That's bad news bears. It's been linked to cognitive decline and even Alzheimer's disease.

By giving your body regular breaks from food, intermittent fasting helps keep insulin levels in check. It's like giving your brain's insulin receptors a chance to breathe and reset. The result? Better cognitive function, reduced risk of neurodegenerative diseases, and a brain that ages like fine wine instead of milk left out on the counter.

Fasting Flexibility: Finding Your Groove

Now, before you start panicking about never eating again, let me reassure you – intermittent fasting comes in many flavors. It's not a one-size-fits-all deal. You've got options, my friend.

There's the 16/8 method, a method where you fast for 16 hours and then eat within an 8-hour timeframe. It's like having a really long overnight fast. For many, this means skipping breakfast and having their first meal around noon.

Or maybe you're more of a 5:2 kind of person. That's where you eat normally for five days a week and drastically reduce calories for two non-consecutive days. It's like giving your gut a couple of spa days each week.

The beauty of intermittent fasting is its flexibility. You can adjust it to fit your lifestyle, your body's needs, and your personal preferences. It's not about starving yourself; it's about finding a rhythm that works for you and your gut-brain axis.

The Adjustment Period: Embrace the Hangry

Let's be real for a moment. Starting an intermittent fasting routine isn't all sunshine and rainbows. Your body's been used to a certain eating schedule, and it might throw a bit of a tantrum when you change things up.

You might feel hungry. You might get a little hangry. Your energy levels might dip. But here's the secret – it's temporary. Your body is incredibly adaptable. Give it time, and it'll not only get used to the new eating pattern but start to thrive on it.

Think of it like training for a marathon. The first few runs are tough, but as you stick with it, your body adapts, and eventually, you're cruising along, feeling like a superhero.

The same goes for intermittent fasting. Push through the initial discomfort, and you'll come out the other side with a gut and brain firing on all cylinders.

The Ripple Effect: Beyond the Gut and Brain

While we've been focusing on the gut-brain connection, the benefits of intermittent fasting ripple out to the rest of your body too. We're talking improved insulin sensitivity, better heart health, reduced inflammation, and even potential anti-aging effects.

It's like giving your entire body a tune-up. Your gut gets a break, your brain gets a boost, and the rest of your body comes along for the ride. It's a holistic approach to health that starts with simply changing when you eat.

The Bottom Line: A Feast for Thought Intermittent fasting isn't just about skipping meals. It's about working with your body's natural rhythms to optimize your gut health, supercharge your brain function, and improve your overall wellbeing. It's a powerful tool in your health arsenal, one that doesn't require fancy equipment or expensive supplements – just a little patience and a willingness to listen to your body.

So, the next time your stomach starts grumbling outside your eating window, remember, you're not just feeling hungry.

You're giving your gut a vacation, your brain a boost, and your body a chance to clean house. And that, my friends, is worth a little growling.

Remember, though, that intermittent fasting isn't for everyone. As with any significant change to your eating habits, it's always a good idea to chat with your healthcare provider, especially if you have any underlying health conditions.

In the end, the journey to optimal gut and brain health is a personal one. Intermittent fasting might be your ticket to cognitive clarity and digestive bliss, or it might be just one tool in your wellness toolbox. The key is to listen to your body, experiment thoughtfully, and find what works best for you.

So, are you ready to give your gut a break and your brain a boost? The fasting feast awaits!

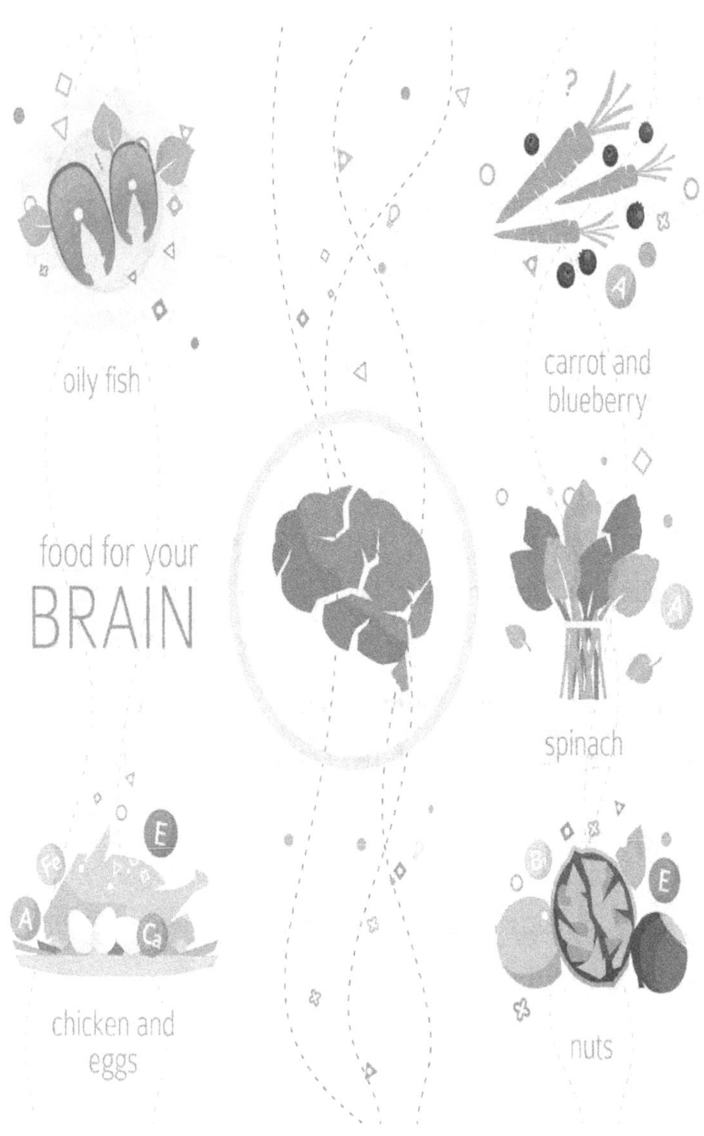

oily fish
carrot and
blueberry
food for your
BRAIN
spinach
chicken and
eggs
nuts

Chapter 4: Real People, Real Results

Real People, Real Results: Gut-Brain Transformations That'll Blow Your Mind

Let's face it, we've all rolled our eyes at those "before and after" stories that sound too good to be true. But buckle up, because the gut-brain connection is about to serve you some truth bombs that'll make you a believer. These aren't your run-of-the-mill success stories – they're raw, real, and might just convince you that your gut has been pulling your mental strings all along.

From Panic to Peace: Sarah Ditches Her Anxiety

Sarah's palms were slick with sweat as she gripped the steering wheel, her heart pounding like a jackhammer in her chest. The familiar sensation of dread washed over her as she sat in gridlocked traffic, late for an important meeting. "Not again," she thought, fighting the urge to abandon her car and flee.

For years, Sarah had been a prisoner of her own mind. Anxiety ruled her life, transforming everyday situations into battlegrounds. Social gatherings felt like minefields, work presentations loomed like executioner's blocks, and even a trip to the grocery store could spiral into a panic attack.

She'd tried it all – therapy, meditation apps, breathing exercises, and even prescription medications. While these tools offered temporary relief, nothing seemed to stick. Sarah felt like she was plugging holes in a sinking ship, always one step away from drowning in her fears.

It wasn't until a chance encounter with a holistic nutritionist at her local farmer's market that Sarah stumbled upon an unexpected path to healing. The nutritionist, noticing Sarah's nervous demeanor, struck up a conversation about the gut-brain connection.

"Your belly and your brain are like best friends who never stop texting," the nutritionist explained, gesturing to her organic produce. "And sometimes, that conversation goes haywire."

Intrigued and desperate for any glimmer of hope, Sarah dove headfirst into researching the gut-brain axis. What she discovered blew her mind: the bustling ecosystem of microbes in her gut wasn't just digesting food – it was pumping out neurotransmitters, influencing her mood, and potentially fueling her anxiety.

Armed with this knowledge, Sarah embarked on a gut-healing journey. She started small, swapping her morning bagel and coffee for a probiotic-rich smoothie bowl. Within days, she noticed subtle shifts – her energy felt more stable, and the constant knot in her stomach began to loosen.

Encouraged, Sarah expanded her gut-friendly arsenal. She experimented with fermented foods, adding tangy sauerkraut to her lunches and discovering a newfound love for kombucha. Prebiotic-rich foods like garlic, onions, and leeks became staples in her cooking, feeding the beneficial bacteria in her gut.

But it wasn't all smooth sailing. Sarah's first attempt at making homemade kefir resulted in a kitchen disaster that left her cat eyeing her suspiciously for days. And convincing herself to try liver pâté – a nutrient powerhouse for gut health – took more willpower than she thought she possessed.

As weeks turned into months, Sarah noticed profound changes. The fog of anxiety that had clouded her mind for years began to lift. She found herself laughing more easily, engaging in conversations without constantly second-guessing herself. Even her sleep improved, with night terrors giving way to restful slumber.

One turning point came during a work presentation. As Sarah stood before her colleagues, she braced herself for the familiar wave of panic. But instead of a tsunami, she felt only a gentle ripple of nerves – manageable, even energizing. She delivered her pitch with confidence, earning praise from her boss and a newfound belief in herself.

Sarah's transformation wasn't limited to her mental state. Her skin cleared up, stubborn digestive issues resolved, and she even shed a few pounds without trying. Friends commented on her newfound glow, asking what her secret was.

"I just started listening to my gut," Sarah would reply with a wink.

Of course, there were challenges along the way. Social situations still required mindful navigation – explaining why she was passing on pizza and beer in favor of a gut-friendly option wasn't always easy. And there were days when old thought patterns tried to creep back in, threatening to undo her progress.

But Sarah had developed a new toolkit. On tough days, she'd whip up a batch of her favorite gut-healing bone broth, letting the aroma fill her kitchen and soothe her senses. She discovered the calming power of chamomile and peppermint teas, using them as a natural alternative to her once-constant anti-anxiety medications.

Perhaps the most profound change was in Sarah's relationship with herself. As she nourished her gut, she learned to extend that same compassion to her mind and spirit. Negative self-talk was replaced with gentle encouragement. She started a gratitude journal, focusing on the small victories each day brought.

Eighteen months into her gut-healing journey, Sarah found herself back in traffic. As horns blared and engines idled, she took a deep breath. Instead of panic, she felt... calm. Reaching into her bag, she pulled out a homemade trail mix of nuts, seeds, and a sprinkle of dark chocolate – her go-to snack for supporting both her gut and her mood.

As she munched, Sarah reflected on how far she'd come. The anxiety that once threatened to swallow her whole had receded to a manageable whisper. She wasn't "cured" – there were still moments of worry, still days when she had to consciously apply her newfound knowledge. But for the first time in years, Sarah felt in control.

Her phone buzzed with a text from a coworker: "Traffic's insane. You're going to be late!"

With a smile, Sarah typed back: "No worries. I've got this."

And she did. Because Sarah had discovered a profound truth – that the path to peace often begins in the most unexpected place: your belly.

Bye-Bye Blues: How Tom Kicked Depression to the Curb

Tom's story begins like many others - a successful career, loving family, and seemingly perfect life on the outside. But behind closed doors, he was fighting a battle that no one could see. Depression had sunk its claws deep into his psyche, turning even the simplest tasks into Herculean efforts.

"I used to wake up feeling like I was wearing a lead suit," Tom recalls, his eyes distant as he remembers those dark days. "Getting out of bed was a victory, showering felt impossible, and forget about being productive at work."

For years, Tom tried the conventional route - therapy, antidepressants, even dabbling in meditation apps that promised instant zen. But nothing seemed to stick. The fog of depression lifted momentarily, only to come crashing back down with a vengeance.

It wasn't until a chance encounter with a nutritionist at his local farmer's market that Tom's journey took an unexpected turn. "She started talking about the gut-brain axis, and honestly, I thought it was some new-age hogwash," Tom chuckles, shaking his head at his former skepticism.

But desperation can be a powerful motivator. With nothing left to lose, Tom decided to give this "gut healing" thing a shot. What followed was a rollercoaster ride of discovery, setbacks, and ultimately, triumph.

The first step? Overhauling his diet. Out went the processed foods, sugary snacks, and late-night pizza binges. In their place came a rainbow of vegetables, fermented foods teeming with probiotics, and omega-3 rich fish that promised to nourish not just his body, but his brain.

"The first week was hell," Tom admits. "I was irritably plagued by headaches, and my family probably wanted to banish me off to a deserted island." But as his body adjusted to this new way of eating, something remarkable began to happen. The fog started to lift, ever so slightly.

Encouraged by these small wins, Tom dove deeper into the world of gut health. He learned about the intricate dance between gut bacteria and neurotransmitters, how inflammation in the gut can trigger inflammation in the brain, and the surprising role that short-chain fatty acids play in mood regulation.

Armed with this knowledge, Tom became his own gut detective. He kept a detailed food and mood journal, tracking how different foods affected his mental state. "I discovered that gluten was my kryptonite," he says. "Every time I ate it, I'd spiral into a funk for days."

But it wasn't just about elimination. Tom also focused on adding in foods that could boost his mood. He became a connoisseur of kefir, experimenting with different flavors and even making his own at home. Prebiotic-rich foods like garlic, onions, and Jerusalem artichokes became staples in his diet, feeding the good bacteria in his gut.

As weeks turned into months, Tom's transformation was nothing short of remarkable. The lead suit he'd been wearing for years seemed to melt away. He found himself waking up before his alarm, eager to start the day. His colleagues noticed a change too - the guy who used to hide in his office was now leading meetings with enthusiasm and cracking jokes by the water cooler.

But perhaps the most significant change was in Tom's relationships. "I was present again," he says, his voice thick with emotion. "I can now actually enjoy quality time with my kids instead of just going through the motions. My wife said it was like getting back the man she fell in love with."

Tom's journey wasn't without its challenges. There were setbacks - a week of travel that threw off his routine, a stressful project at work that tempted him back to his old eating habits. But armed with his new knowledge and a support system that understood the importance of gut health, Tom was able to course-correct quickly.

One of the most surprising aspects of Tom's recovery was how it sparked a ripple effect in his community. Friends and family, intrigued by his transformation, started asking questions. Tom found himself sharing gut health tips at barbecues, swapping fermentation recipes with neighbors, and even starting a small support group for others struggling with depression.

"It's not just about the food," Tom explains. "It's about understanding that our bodies are these incredible, interconnected systems. When you start treating your gut with respect, it's like you're finally speaking the same language as your body."

Today, Tom is not just depression-free - he's thriving in ways he never thought possible. He's taken up rock climbing, started a podcast about mental health and nutrition, and is even writing a cookbook filled with gut-friendly comfort foods.

"I'm not saying gut health is a magic bullet for everyone," Tom cautions. "But for me, I can happily say it was the key that unlocked a door I thought was shut permanently. Depression isn't just 'in your head' - it's in your gut, your diet, your lifestyle. And when you address all of those pieces, that's when real healing can begin."

As our interview winds down, Tom's eyes sparkle with a vitality that was once lost to the depths of depression. He leans in, as if sharing a secret, and says, "You know, I used to think happiness was this elusive thing that happened to other people. Now I am certain it all starts in the gut. And let me tell you, a happy gut makes for one happy human."

Tom's story is a powerful testament to the transformative potential of the gut-brain axis. It reminds us that sometimes, the path to mental wellness doesn't just lie in our minds, but in the complex ecosystem thriving within our bellies. For those still struggling in the shadows of depression, Tom's journey offers a glimmer of hope - that with the right knowledge, support, and a lot of fermented foods, it's possible to not just say goodbye to the blues, but to embrace a life filled with color, joy, and endless possibilities.

Gut-Brain Success Stories from Real People Like You

Ever felt like you were the only one struggling with mysterious mood swings, brain fog that wouldn't lift, or anxiety that came out of nowhere? Well, buckle up, because you're about to meet some folks who've been right where you are – and found their way out through the power of gut health. These aren't polished celebrity stories or carefully crafted marketing tales. These are real people, just like you and me, who stumbled upon the gut-brain connection and decided to give it a shot. Get ready for some raw, honest, and downright inspiring journeys that'll make you think, "Hey, if they can do it, maybe I can too!"

Meet Jake: From Couch Potato to Marathon Man

Jake was your typical 30-something office worker, living on energy drinks and takeout. He'd drag himself to work, zone out at his desk, and come home too exhausted to do much beyond binge-watching TV. Weekends? Those were for recovering from the work week.

"I just thought being tired and cranky all the time was part of being an adult," Jake admits with a laugh. "Boy, was I wrong."

It was a chance conversation with a health-nut coworker that put gut health on Jake's radar. Skeptical but desperate, he decided to give it a try. He started small, swapping his morning energy drink for a probiotic-rich smoothie and his lunchtime burger for a colorful salad with fermented veggies.

"The first week was rough," Jake remembers. "I was grumpy, and I swear I could hear my gut rumbling in discomfort. But by week two, something shifted. I woke up one Saturday and actually wanted to go for a walk. Me! The guy who considered the distance from the couch to the fridge a workout!"

Fast forward six months, and Jake's life is barely recognizable. He's running 5Ks, meal prepping like a pro, and even signed up for his first half-marathon.

"The best part? My mind feels clear for the first time in years. I'm killing it at work, I'm present in my relationships, and I actually look forward to my days. Who knew your gut could change so much?"

Samantha's Story: Silencing the Anxiety Alarm
Samantha was the person everyone dubbed "high-strung." A successful lawyer with a picture-perfect life on paper, she was constantly battling an inner storm of worry and panic.

"I'd wake up at 3 AM in a cold sweat, my mind racing with worst-case scenarios," Samantha shares. "Meditation, therapy, medication – I tried it all. Nothing seemed to quiet that constant alarm in my head."

It was during a particularly bad bout of IBS that Samantha first heard about the gut-brain axis. Desperate for relief from her physical symptoms, she dove headfirst into researching the connection.

"I overhauled my diet completely," she explains. "I gave up junk food and late-night wine. In came bone broth, kimchi, and more veggies than I knew what to do with. I even started fermenting my own kombucha – me, the takeout queen!"

The change wasn't overnight, but it was undeniable. Within a month, Samantha noticed she was sleeping through the night more often. By month three, she was handling high-stress court cases with a newfound calm.

"Don't get me wrong, I still get nervous once in a while," Samantha clarifies. "But it's normal nervous, not that very overwhelming wave of anxiety. For the first time in my life, I feel like I'm in control of my emotions, not the other way around."

The Unlikely Gut Health Convert: Mike's Journey from Skeptic to Believer

Mike was the guy who rolled his eyes at every new health trend. A retired mechanic with a love for classic cars and classic American food, he wasn't about to start eating "rabbit food" or drinking weird fermented teas.

"I thought all this gut health stuff was a bunch of hogwash," Mike admits gruffly. "But when you've been feeling lousy for years and the doctors can't figure out why, you get desperate enough to try anything."

Mike's main complaints were constant fatigue, joint pain, and a fog that made it hard to focus on his beloved car restorations. His daughter, worried about her dad's declining health, finally convinced him to see a functional medicine doctor who specialized in gut health.

"I went in there ready to argue," Mike chuckles. "But this doc, she listened. Really listened. And then she explained how all the junk I was eating was basically declaring war on my gut, and my gut was fighting back by messing with the rest of my body."

Reluctantly, Mike agreed to a 30-day gut reset protocol. No gluten, no dairy, no processed foods. Lots of vegetables, lean proteins, and yes, even some of that weird fermented stuff.

"The first two weeks were hell," Mike admits. "I was grumpy, I had headaches, and I swear I even dream about cheeseburgers. But then something strange happened. I woke up one morning and realized... nothing hurt. My joints weren't aching. My head felt clear."

By the end of the 30 days, Mike was a changed man. His energy was through the roof, he was sleeping better than he had in decades, and he even lost the spare tire around his middle.

"I won't lie, I still miss a good pizza now and then," Mike says. "But feeling this good? It's worth giving up a few things. Plus, my grandkids are thrilled that Grandpa can get down on the floor and play with them now."

The Teenage Turnaround: Zoe's Battle with Depression

Zoe's story reminds us that gut health isn't just for adults. This vibrant 17-year-old went from barely being able to get out of bed to becoming a mental health advocate in her school.

"It started in freshman year," Zoe recalls. "I just felt... heavy. Like this dark cloud was following me everywhere. I lost interest in everything – my friends, my hobbies, even my favorite foods."

Zoe's parents were terrified. They tried therapy, medications, even a brief hospitalization. While these interventions helped, Zoe still felt like she was viewing life through a gray filter.

It was a chance encounter with a holistic nutritionist at a health fair that put Zoe on the path to healing. The nutritionist explained how the standard American teenage diet – full of sugar, processed foods, and artificial everything

– could be wreaking havoc on Zoe's gut and, by extension, her brain.

"I was skeptical at first," Zoe admits. "I mean, how could changing what I eat have an impact on my depression? But at that point I was willing to try just anything."

Zoe and her family embarked on a gut-healing journey together. They cleared out the pantry, learned to cook healing foods, and even started a small vegetable garden in their backyard.

"The coolest part was learning about all these foods I'd never tried before," Zoe enthuses. "Like, who knew there were so many varieties of mushrooms? Or that sauerkraut could actually taste good?"

As Zoe's diet changed, so did her mood. The fog began to lift. Colors seemed brighter. She found herself laughing at jokes again, wanting to hang out with friends.

"It wasn't a magic cure," Zoe says. Frankly speaking, "I still see my therapist, and some days are harder than others. But now I have this toolkit of foods and habits that I know will support my mental health. It's like I finally found the instruction manual for my body and brain."

Today, Zoe is passionate about spreading the word about gut health to other teens. She started a "Happy Gut Club" at her high school, where students learn about nutrition, cook healthy meals together, and support each other's mental health journeys.

"If I can at least help even one other kid feel better, then it's worth it," Zoe says with a smile. "Plus, my mom says I'm teaching her new recipes now, which is pretty cool."

These stories are just a small sample of the countless lives transformed by the power of gut health. From busy professionals to skeptical retirees to struggling teenagers, the gut-brain connection has the potential to revolutionize how we approach mental and physical well-being.

Remember, everyone's journey is unique. What works for one person may not have the same effect on another. But these stories show us that there's hope, that feeling better is possible, and that sometimes, the key to a healthier mind might just be hiding in your belly.

So, are you ready to write your own gut-brain success story?

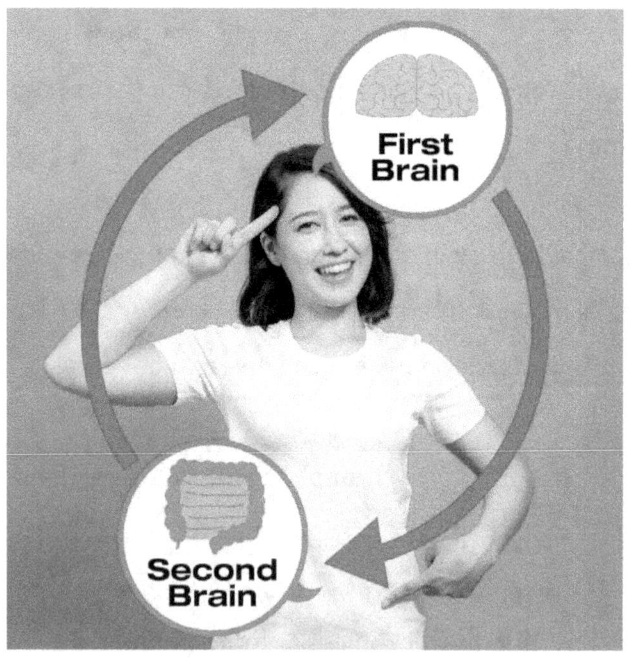

Chapter 5: The Nerdy (but Exciting) Stuff

Hey there, brain-hackers and gut-enthusiasts! Ready to geek out with me? Don't worry, I promise to keep things spicy – we're talking about your second brain, after all!

Mind-Blowing New Research: What Scientists Are Discovering About Your Gut

Picture this: a bustling city of trillions, all working in harmony (mostly) to keep you thinking straight and feeling great. That's your gut microbiome, and scientists are uncovering new secrets about it every day.

Did you know that your gut bacteria have a day job and a night shift? Yep, recent studies show that your microbiome follows a circadian rhythm, just like you do. This discovery is huge because it means that when you eat could be just as important as what you eat when it comes to keeping your gut-brain axis humming.

But wait, there's more! Researchers at the University of California, Los Angeles, found that certain gut bacteria can actually predict how your brain will react to different foods. It's like having a tiny fortune teller in your belly!

And here's a wild one: scientists at the APC Microbiome Ireland institute discovered that some gut bacteria produce tiny, molecule-sized "spaceships" called extracellular vesicles. These little guys can cross the blood-brain barrier and directly influence your brain cells. Talk about a long-distance relationship!

The Future Is Now: Personalized Gut Hacks for Your Unique Brain

Buckle up, because the future of gut-brain health is looking like a sci-fi movie – in the best way possible.

Imagine popping into your local pharmacy for a quick gut check. You spit in a tube, and within minutes, a machine analyzes your unique microbiome composition. Based on the results, it prints out a personalized diet plan and probiotic prescription tailored specifically to your gut's needs. Sounds far-fetched? Well, companies like DayTwo and Viome are already offering similar services, and the technology is only getting better.

But why stop there? Researchers are working on "psychobiotics" – specific strains of bacteria that could be used to treat mental health conditions. Feeling anxious?

There might be a bacterial cocktail for that in the near future. And for all you tech-lovers out there, how about a smart toilet that analyzes your, ahem, donations to science every day?

MIT researchers are developing just that. It could alert you to any changes in your microbiome and suggest dietary tweaks before problems arise. Talk about a helpful throne!

Straight Talk: Interviews with Gut-Brain Gurus

I sat down with some of the brightest minds in the gut-brain field, and let me tell you, these conversations were mind-bending. Here are some highlights:

Dr. Emeran Mayer, author of "The Mind-Gut Connection", dropped this bomb: "We're discovering that the gut microbiome might play a role in how we form memories. Certain bacteria seem to influence the production of proteins crucial for memory formation."

I nearly fell off my chair when Dr. Kirsten Tillisch, a pioneering researcher in the field, told me, "We're seeing evidence that the gut microbiome could influence personality traits. It's early days, but the implications are staggering."

And get this – Dr. John Cryan, who's been studying the gut-brain axis for over a decade, shared an insight that blew my mind: "We're finding that the vagus nerve, which connects the gut to the brain, might be more of a two-way street than we thought.

Your thoughts and emotions could be influencing your gut bacteria just as much as they're influencing you."

But it's not all lab coats and petri dishes. I also chatted with Sandor Katz, the fermentation guru behind "Wild Fermentation". He reminded me that some of the most powerful gut-brain medicines are sitting in your kitchen right now.

"Every culture has its own traditional fermented foods," he said. "These time-tested recipes are like a direct line to our ancestral microbiome."

The Gut-Brain Axis: Where Science Meets Science Fiction

As we wrap up our nerdy (but oh-so-exciting) journey, let's take a moment to appreciate just how wild this all is. We're not just talking about eating better to feel better – we're talking about a paradigm shift in how we understand the very essence of who we are.

Think about it: every thought you have, every emotion you feel, might be influenced by the trillions of tiny creatures living in your gut. And in turn, your thoughts and feelings are shaping their world.

It's a beautiful, symbiotic dance that's been going on since the dawn of humanity, and we're only just now learning the steps.

But here's the really exciting part, armed with this knowledge, you have more power than ever to shape your mental and emotional well-being.

Every meal is an opportunity to nourish not just your body, but your mind. Every new habit is a chance to cultivate a healthier, happier gut community.

As we stand on the brink of this gut-brain revolution, one thing is clear, the future of mental health is in your hands or rather, in your belly. So go forth, experiment, and listen to your gut. It has more to say than you might think!

Conclusion: Your No-B.S. Guide to Lasting Brain Bliss

If you've found value in this book, I'd be immensely grateful if you could leave a review. Your feedback not only helps me improve but also guides others on their path to gut-brain health. Together we can spark a gut-brain revolution!

Alright, let's wrap this gut-brain adventure up with a bang! Here's your no-nonsense guide to keeping that brain of yours in tip-top shape:

Listen up, because this is where the conversation gets real. We've been on quite a journey, haven't we? From discovering that second brain lurking in your belly to learning how to feed those trillions of tiny mood managers. But now it's time to put it all together and create your personalized blueprint for lasting brain bliss.

First things first: there's no one-size-fits-all solution here. Your gut is as unique as your fingerprint, and what works for your bestie might not work for you. But that's the beauty of this whole gut-brain connection – you get to be the scientist of your own body.

Remember when we talked about how your gut influences everything from your stress levels to your ability to focus? Well, now it's time to take that knowledge and run with it. Think of your newfound gut wisdom as your secret weapon against the chaos of everyday life.

Let's break it down into actionable steps, shall we?

1. Tune in to your gut feelings – literally. Notice how different foods influence how you feel. That bloated, foggy feeling after your favorite greasy burger? Yeah, that's your gut trying to tell you something.

2. Embrace the power of variety. Your gut microbes are like a picky audience – they want to be entertained with a diverse menu. So, mix it up! Try that strange but intriguing vegetable at the farmer's market. Your gut bugs might just throw a party.

3. Stress less, digest better. Remember how we talked about the stress-gut connection? Time to put some relaxation techniques into practice. Maybe it's yoga, maybe it's belting out show tunes in the shower – find what works for you.

4. Sleep like your brain depends on it – because it does. We didn't dive too deep into sleep before, but trust me, it's crucial for both your gut and your brain. Aim for those solid 7-9 hours.

5. Move that body! Exercise isn't just for your muscles. It's a VIP pass for your gut microbes to thrive. Find something you enjoy, whether it's dancing, hiking, or chasing your dog around the yard.

6. Stay hydrated, my friends. Water is the secret weapon for a healthy gut. It keeps things moving, if you know what I mean.

7. Embrace fermented foods. They're like a probiotic party in your mouth. Kimchi, kombucha, kefir – experiment and find your favorites.

8. Don't forget your fiber. It's like a broom for your insides, keeping everything clean and your gut bugs happy.

9. Cut back on the processed junk. Your gut microbes are not fans of artificial additives and preservatives. Neither is your brain, for that matter.

10. Be patient and persistent. Rome wasn't built in a day, and neither is a healthy gut-brain axis. Give it time, and don't beat yourself up if you slip up now and then.

Now, let's talk about the long game. This isn't just about feeling good for a few weeks. It's about creating a lifestyle that supports your brain health for years to come.

Imagine waking up every day feeling clear-headed and ready to tackle whatever life throws at you. Picture yourself navigating stressful situations with ease, your mood steady as a rock. That's the power of a well-tuned gut-brain axis.

But here's the kicker, this journey doesn't end with the last page of this book. Science is constantly evolving, and new discoveries about the gut-brain connection are being made all the time. Stay curious, consistent learning, and don't be afraid to try new delicacies.

Remember those success stories we shared earlier? Those could be you. But it's going to take more than just wishful thinking. It's going to take action, consistency, and a willingness to listen to your body.

So, what's your next move? Maybe it's clearing out your pantry and restocking it with gut-friendly foods. Perhaps it's finally signing up for that meditation class you've been eyeing. Or it could be as simple as swapping your morning coffee for a gut-loving green smoothie.

Whatever it is, take that first step. Your future self will thank you for it. Because here's the truth – a happy gut leads to a happy brain, and a happy brain leads to a happier, healthier you.

You've got the knowledge, you've got the tools, and now you've got a roadmap. The rest is up to you. So go forth and conquer, gut warrior. Your brain bliss awaits!

And hey, if you ever feel lost or overwhelmed, flip back through these pages. Let them be your guide, your cheerleader, and your reminder of why you started this journey in the first place.

Here's to your gut, your brain, and the amazing connection between them. May your microbiome flourish, your neurons fire with joy, and your life be filled with the kind of vitality that comes from true gut-brain harmony.

Now, go out there and show the world what a gut-brain superhero looks like. Trust me, it looks a lot like you.

Bonus Goodies:

Alright, fellow gut-brain explorers, it's time to raid the grocery store like it's Black Friday for your belly! But instead of fighting over the last flat-screen TV, we're going to load up on nature's brain-boosters. Buckle up, because this isn't your grandma's shopping list – unless your grandma was secretly a neuroscientist with a penchant for fermented foods.

Gut-Brain All-Stars: Your Shopping List for a Happy Mind

1. The Omega-3 Ocean Squad

First stop: the seafood section. We're talking wild-caught salmon, sardines, and mackerel. These fatty fish are swimming in omega-3s, the brain's favorite building blocks. Can't stand the smell of fish? No worries! Grab some walnuts, chia seeds, or flaxseeds instead. They're like little omega-3 grenades, ready to explode with brain-boosting goodness.

2. The Probiotic Party Animals

Next up, we're hitting the fermented food aisle. Kimchi, sauerkraut, kefir, and kombucha – these aren't just trendy hipster foods, they're teeming with beneficial bacteria that'll turn your gut into a five-star hotel for good microbes. And trust me, when your gut bugs are happy, your brain throws a party.

3. The Fiber Fanatics

Let's not forget about prebiotics – the food for your good gut bacteria. Load up on Jerusalem artichokes, garlic, onions, leeks, asparagus, and bananas. These fiber-rich foods are like an all-you-can-eat buffet for your microbiome. Your gut bugs will be so grateful, they might just help you remember where you left your keys.

4. The Antioxidant A-Team

Blueberries, blackberries, raspberries – oh my! These little flavor bombs are packed with antioxidants that fight inflammation faster than a superhero takes down a villain. Throw in some dark chocolate (yes, really!) and you've got a brain-protecting powerhouse that also satisfies your sweet tooth. Talk about a win-win!

5. The Leafy Green League

Kale, spinach, Swiss chard – if it's green and leafy, throw it in your cart. These nutrient-dense superstars are loaded with vitamins, minerals, and phytonutrients that your brain craves. Plus, they're versatile enough to sneak into smoothies if you're not a salad fan. Popeye was onto something with his spinach obsession, folks.

6. The Spice Rack Rebels

Don't sleep on your spices! Turmeric, with its active compound curcumin, is like a golden ticket to reduced inflammation. Pair it with black pepper to boost absorption. Cinnamon isn't just for lattes – it can help balance blood sugar, which is crucial for brain health. And rosemary? It's not just for roast chicken; it's been shown to boost memory and concentration.

7. The Nutty Professors

Almonds, cashews, pistachios – these aren't just for squirrels. Nuts are packed with vitamin E, healthy fats, and minerals that your brain adores. They're like little helmets for your neurons. Just remember, a handful is plenty – we're aiming for brain food, not a food baby.

8. The Avocado Avengers

Avocados deserve their own category. These creamy green gods are packed with monounsaturated fats that help maintain healthy blood flow – and your brain loves a good blood flow. Smash them on toast, blend them into smoothies, or eat them straight with a spoon (we won't judge).

9. The Egg-cellent Brainiacs

Eggs are like nature's multivitamin. The yolks are rich in choline, a nutrient crucial for brain health that most of us don't get enough of. They're also packed with B vitamins, which help produce neurotransmitters. Forget which came first – the chicken or the egg and just get both in your cart.

10. The Bone Broth Brigade

Don't knock it 'til you've tried it! Bone broth is rich in collagen, amino acids, and minerals that support gut health. It's like a warm hug for your intestines. Plus, it's versatile –

use it as a base for soups, sauces, or sip it straight when you're feeling fancy.

11. The Cruciferous Crusaders

Broccoli, cauliflower, Brussels sprouts – these might have been your childhood nemesis, but they're your adult brain's BFF. They're packed with sulforaphane, a compound that's been shown to have neuroprotective properties. Roast them, steam them, or sneak them into a stir-fry – just get them in your belly!

12. The Purple Powerhouses

Eggplant, purple cabbage, purple potatoes – if it's purple, it's probably packed with anthocyanins, powerful antioxidants that give these foods their vibrant color. These compounds have been linked to improved memory and reduced risk of cognitive decline. Plus, they make your plate look like a work of art.

13. The Olive Oil Operators

Extra virgin olive oil isn't just for fancy salad dressings. It's rich in polyphenols, compounds that protect your brain cells from damage. Drizzle it on everything – your brain (and taste buds) will thank you.

14. The Mushroom Magicians

Lion's mane, reishi, shiitake – these fungi are having a moment, and for good reason. They're packed with compounds that support brain health, reduce inflammation, and may even help grow new brain cells. Add them to soups, stir-fries, or steep them in tea for a brain-boosting brew.

15. The Seed Saviors

Pumpkin seeds, sunflower seeds, hemp seeds – these little powerhouses are packed with zinc, magnesium, and omega-3s. Sprinkle them on salads, blend them into smoothies, or just munch on them when you need a brain-boosting snack.

Remember, this isn't just a shopping list – it's your ticket to a happier, healthier brain. But here's the kicker: it's not about perfection. You don't need to buy everything on this list every week (unless you've got a pantry the size of a small country). Start small, experiment, and find what works for you.

And hey, if you find yourself staring at the kombucha section wondering if you've lost your mind, just remember – your gut bugs are cheering you on. They're like tiny cheerleaders in your belly, doing backflips every time you choose brain-boosting foods.

So go forth, brave gut-brain warriors, and conquer that grocery store. Your mind (and your microbiome) will thank you. And who knows? Maybe the next time you're looking for your keys, they'll be right where you left them – imagine that!

Too Busy to Cook? Quick Recipes for Gut-Brain Goodness

Let's face it - we're all living life in the fast lane these days. Between work, family, and trying to squeeze in a social life, who has time to spend hours in the kitchen whipping up gourmet meals? But here's the kicker - your gut (and by extension, your brain) doesn't care about your busy schedule. It needs good food, and it needs it now.

Don't worry, I've got your back. As someone who once thought a balanced meal was a coffee in each hand, I've learned the hard way that quick doesn't have to mean unhealthy. So, let's dive into some lightning-fast recipes that'll make your gut sing and your brain do a happy dance.

1. The "morning rush-hour" Breakfast Smoothie

Time: 5 minutes

Ingredients:

- 1 cup unsweetened almond milk
- 1 handful of spinach (trust me, you won't taste it)
- 1 banana
- 1 tablespoon almond butter
- 1 scoop of your preferred protein powder
- 1 teaspoon chia seeds
- Ice cubes

Toss it all into a blender, hit the button, and voila! You've got a nutrient-packed breakfast that'll keep your gut bugs happy and your brain firing on all cylinders. The spinach provides fiber for your gut microbiome, while the banana offers prebiotics. The almond butter and chia seeds give you a dose of omega-3s, which your brain absolutely loves.

2. The "My Lunch Break Is Way Too Short" Salad Jar

Time: 10 minutes (prep night before, eat whenever)

Ingredients:

- Mason jar

- 2 tablespoons olive oil and balsamic vinegar dressing

- 1/4 cup cherry tomatoes, halved

- 1/4 cup cucumber, diced

- 1/4 cup chickpeas

- 1/4 avocado, cubed

- Handful of mixed greens

- 2 tablespoons pumpkin seeds

Layer these ingredients in the order listed (dressing at the bottom, greens at the top). When hunger strikes, just shake it up and dig in.

The chickpeas and avocado provide fiber and healthy fats, while the pumpkin seeds offer zinc and omega-3s - all great for your gut-brain axis.

3. The "I Can't Be Bothered to Cook" Dinner Bowl

Time: 15 minutes

Ingredients:

- 1 cup cooked quinoa (make a big batch on weekends)

- 1/2 cup roasted vegetables (whatever's in your fridge)

- 1/4 cup hummus

- 1/4 avocado, sliced

- Handful of spinach

- 1 tablespoon olive oil

- Squeeze of lemon

- Pinch of sea salt and pepper

Mix it all in a bowl and enjoy. Quinoa is a complete protein and packed with fiber. The roasted veggies provide a variety of nutrients, while the hummus offers more fiber and healthy fats. It's a gut-brain party in a bowl!

4. The "Netflix and Chill" Snack Attack

Time: 2 minutes

Ingredients:

- 1 cup plain Greek yogurt

- 1/4 cup mixed berries

- 1 tablespoon honey

- 1 tablespoon chopped walnuts

Layer in a glass or bowl for a fancy touch. The Greek yogurt is loaded with probiotics for your gut, berries provide antioxidants for your brain, and walnuts offer omega-3s. It's like ice cream, but your gut and brain will thank you.

5. The "I Need Comfort Food" Soup

Time: 20 minutes

Ingredients:

- 4 cups bone broth (store-bought is fine)

- 1 cup mixed vegetables (frozen is okay)

- 1 cup cooked shredded chicken

- 1 teaspoon turmeric

- 1 teaspoon ginger

- Salt and pepper to taste

Simmer everything together and enjoy. Bone broth is fantastic for gut health, providing collagen and amino acids. Turmeric and ginger are anti-inflammatory superstars that your gut and brain will love.

Remember, feeding your gut-brain axis doesn't have to be complicated or time-consuming. It's about making creative choices with your time. These recipes are just the beginning - feel free to experiment and find what works for you.

Pro tip: Prep ingredients in bulk when you do have time. Chop veggies, cook grains, and prepare proteins in advance. Future-you will be grateful when you're knee-deep in a busy week.

Listen, I get it. When life gets hectic, it's tempting to reach for that takeout menu or pop a frozen dinner in the microwave. But think of your gut as your internal best friend. It's always there for you, working hard to keep you healthy and happy. The least we can do is throw it a bone (or a quick, nutritious meal) every now and then.

Remember, every bite is an opportunity to nourish your gut and, by extension, your brain. So, the next time you think you're too busy to cook, give one of these recipes a shot. Your gut will thank you, your brain will high-five you, and who knows? You might just find yourself with more energy to tackle that to-do list.

Supplement Savvy: What to Take for Your Tummy and Noggin

Let's face it, folks – navigating the wild world of supplements can feel like trying to decipher ancient hieroglyphics while riding a unicycle. Blindfolded. But fear not! I'm about to break it down for you in a way that'll make you feel like a gut-brain guru in no time.

First things first: supplements aren't magic pills. They're more like the backup dancers to the lead singer that is your diet. Important? Absolutely. The whole show? Not quite. But when you get the right ones, oh boy, can they make your gut and brain sing in harmony!

The Probiotic Parade

Let's kick things off with probiotics – the tiny superheroes of your gut. These little guys are like a peacekeeping force for your intestines, keeping the bad bugs in check and the good vibes flowing. But here's the kicker: not all probiotics are created equal.

Look for strains like Lactobacillus and Bifidobacterium. They're the cool kids on the probiotic block. And don't just grab any old bottle off the shelf. Aim for at least 10 billion CFUs (that's Colony Forming Units for you science nerds out there). Oh, and make sure they've got a variety of strains. Your gut likes diversity – think of it as a microbial melting pot.

Omega-3s: The Brain's Best Friend

Next up, we've got omega-3 fatty acids. DHA and EPA, the two rock stars of the omega-3 world, are crucial for keeping your noggin in tip-top shape. They help with everything from mood regulation to memory.

But here's a little secret: your body can't make these on its own. It's like trying to bake a cake without flour (ain't gonna happen). So unless you're chowing down on salmon every day (and let's be real, who is?), an omega-3 supplement might be your ticket to brain town.

Look for a high-quality fish oil supplement or, if you're plant-based, algae-based omega-3s. And don't skimp on the dosage – aim for at least 1000mg of combined EPA and DHA daily. Your brain cells will be doing a happy dance, trust me.

The Magnificent Magnesium

Now, let's talk about the unsung hero of the supplement world: magnesium. This mineral is like the Swiss Army knife of nutrients. It's involved in over 300 enzymatic reactions in your body. That's right, 300! It's crucial for everything from sleep to stress management. most of us are walking around magnesium deficient and don't even know it. It's like having a superpower and not actually being aware. Tragic, really.

When shopping for magnesium, look for magnesium glycinate or magnesium threonate. They're more easily absorbed and less likely to give you, ahem, digestive surprises. Start with about 200-400mg daily and see how you feel. You might just find yourself sleeping like a baby and handling stress like a zen master.

Vitamin D: The Sunshine Supplement

Alright, let's shine a light on vitamin D. This isn't just for strong bones, folks. Vitamin D is a crucial player in the gut-brain game. It helps regulate the immune system, reduces inflammation, and even plays a role in mood regulation.

Here's the thing: unless you're a lizard sunbathing on a rock all day, you're probably not getting enough. And no, sitting by a window doesn't count. Your body needs direct sunlight to make vitamin D.

Aim for about 1000-2000 IU daily, but here's a pro tip: get your levels checked first. Vitamin D is fat-soluble, which means it can build up in your body. You want the Goldilocks amount – not too little, not too much, but just right.

The Adaptogen All-Stars

Now, let's venture into the world of adaptogens. These aren't your average supplements. They're like nature's chill pills, helping your body adapt to stress. And let's face it, in today's world, we could all use a little help in the stress department.

Two adaptogens to keep on your radar: Ashwagandha and Rhodiola. Ashwagandha is like a warm hug for your nervous system. It can help reduce cortisol (that pesky stress hormone) and may even improve sleep quality.

Rhodiola, on the other hand, is like a gentle energy boost without the jitters. It can help combat fatigue and improve mental performance. Just imagine tackling your to-do list with the focus of a Zen master and the energy of a caffeinated squirrel. That's Rhodiola for you.

Start with about 300mg of Ashwagandha or 200mg of Rhodiola daily. But remember, adaptogens work best when you're consistent. Give them a few weeks to really see the magic happen.

The B-vitamin Bonanza

Last but certainly not least, let's talk B-vitamins. These guys are like the backstage crew at a rock concert – you don't see them, but boy, do they keep the show running smoothly.

B-vitamins are crucial for energy production, nerve function, and even the production of neurotransmitters (those chemical messengers in your brain). But here's the catch: they're water-soluble, which means your body doesn't store them. You need a constant supply.

Look for a B-complex that includes all eight B-vitamins. Pay special attention to B12, folate, and B6 – they're particularly important for brain health. And if you're plant-based, listen up: you might need to supplement with B12, as it's mainly found in animal products.

The Supplement Symphony

Now, before you rush off to buy out the entire supplement aisle, remember this: supplements work best as part of a balanced approach. They're not a replacement for a healthy diet, good sleep, and regular exercise. Think of them as the cherry on top of your wellness sundae.

And here's a crucial point: not all supplements play nice together. Some can interact with medications or even cancel each other out. It's like inviting your ex and your current partner to the same party – things could get messy.

Always, and I mean always, chat with a healthcare professional before starting any new supplement regimen. They can help you create a personalized plan that's tailored to your unique needs. It's like having a personal stylist for your insides!

The Bottom Line

Supplements can be powerful allies in your gut-brain health journey. But remember, they're called supplements for a reason – they're meant to supplement a healthy lifestyle, not replace it.

Begin with small steps, be consistent, and tune in to your body. It might take some trial and error to find the right combination for you. But when you do? Oh boy, it's like finding the perfect pair of jeans – everything just fits.

So go forth, my gut-brain warriors! Armed with this knowledge, you're ready to navigate the supplement aisle like a pro. Your tummy and noggin will thank you. And who knows? You might just become the go-to guru in your friend group for all things gut and brain. Now wouldn't that be something to digest?

On-the-Go Gut Health Hacks: Because Life Doesn't Stop for Your Belly

Let's face it - life moves at breakneck speed. Between juggling work, family, and that ever-elusive "me time," it's easy to let your gut health slide. But here's the kicker: your belly doesn't take a day off, even when you're running on fumes. So, how do you keep your gut happy when you're living life in the fast lane? Buckle up, buttercup - we're about to dive into some game-changing gut health hacks that'll fit into even the busiest of schedules.

1. The Mindful Munch

You're scarfing down lunch at your desk, eyes glued to your screen, barely tasting your food. Sound familiar? Let's hit the brakes on this habit. Enter: the mindful munch. Take just five minutes to step away from your work, focus on your meal, and chew slowly. It's not rocket science, but its amazingly effective. Your gut will thank you for the extra time to process, and bonus - you might actually enjoy your food for once!

2. Hydration Station

Water might not be sexy, but it's your gut's secret weapon. Keep a reusable water bottle with you at all times - make it your new fashion accessory if you have to. Aim to sip throughout the day, not chug. Your gut microbes love a well-hydrated environment, and you'll be amazed at how much better you feel when you're not running on empty.

3. Stress-Busting Breathing

Stuck in traffic? Feeling the pressure before a big meeting? Time for some belly breathing. Place one hand on your stomach, inhale deeply through your nose for four counts, hold for seven, then exhale for eight.

This little trick activates your parasympathetic nervous system, telling your body it's time to "rest and digest" rather than "fight or flight." Your gut and your mind will both simmer down.

4. The Probiotic Purse Stash

Keeping your good gut bugs happy doesn't have to mean lugging around a cooler of yogurt. Stash some shelf-stable probiotic supplements in your bag, car, or desk drawer. Pop one when you feel your digestion needs a boost, like after that greasy fast-food lunch you instantly regretted.

5. The Fiber Find

Fiber is your gut's BFF, but it doesn't always come in the most convenient packages. Enter: portable fiber options. Toss some nuts, seeds, or dried fruit into a small container for an on-the-go fiber fix. Or, if you're feeling fancy, whip up some homemade energy balls packed with oats, chia seeds, and dried fruit. Your gut will do a happy dance, and your taste buds won't complain either.

6. The Standing Solution

Sitting is the new smoking, they say. But who has time for hour-long walks when deadlines are looming? Try this: stand up every hour, even if it's just for a minute or two. Do a few stretches, march in place, or if you're feeling brave, throw in some squats. This mini-movement break gets your blood flowing, which in turn keeps your gut moving. It's a win-win for your body and your productivity.

7. The Herbal Helper

Green tea isn't just for zen moments at home. Pack some tea bags in your bag and ask for hot water wherever you go. Green tea is packed with polyphenols that your gut microbes love to munch on. Plus, the ritual of sipping tea can be a mindful moment in your chaotic day.

8. The Gut-Friendly Snack Attack

When hunger strikes and the vending machine beckons, be prepared with gut-friendly snacks. Think apple slices with almond butter, carrot sticks with hummus, or a small handful of mixed nuts and seeds. These options offer a mix of fiber, healthy fats, and proteins that'll keep both you and your gut bacteria satisfied.

9. The Power of Fermentation

Fermented foods are like a party for your gut microbes. While you can't exactly carry around a jar of kimchi (or maybe you can, no judgment here), there are portable options. Try some dried nori sheets for a salty, umami-rich snack that's packed with gut-loving compounds. Or, if you're feeling adventurous, give fermented protein bars a try - they're becoming increasingly popular and offer a probiotic punch.

10. The Massage Moment

Stuck in a long meeting or on a never-ending conference call? Here's a stealth move: give yourself a quick abdominal massage. Use your fingertips to make gentle circular motions around your belly button, moving outward. This can help stimulate digestion and relieve tension. Just try not to make it too obvious - your coworkers might start to wonder what you're up to!

11. The Posture Check

Your posture affects your gut more than you might think. Set a reminder on your phone to do a posture check every couple of hours. Stand tall, roll back your shoulders, and breathe in fully. This simple adjustment can improve digestion and reduce bloating. Plus, you'll look more confident - fake it 'til you make it, right?

12. The Zen Zone

Create a "zen zone" wherever you go. It could be as simple as a calming playlist on your phone or a few drops of lavender essential oil on a handkerchief. When stress hits (and let's face it, it will), take a moment to breathe deeply and engage with your zen tool of choice. Remember, a calm mind leads to a calmer gut.

13. The Gut-Brain Check-In

Last but not least, practice regular gut-brain check-ins. Take a moment to pause and ask yourself: How does my gut feel right now? Am I bloated? Gassy? Comfortable? This mindfulness practice helps you tune into your body's signals and make adjustments as needed.

Remember, these hacks aren't about perfection - they're about progress. Your gut is as unique as you are, so what works for your coworker might not work for you.

Experiment, have fun with it, and most importantly, listen to your body. It's got a lot to say if you're willing to listen.

So, the next time life throws you a curveball (or a dozen), you'll be armed with these gut-friendly strategies. Because while life doesn't stop for your belly, with these hacks, it doesn't have to. Here's to happy guts and healthier minds, no matter where your day takes you!